SUPER PLANT-BASED RECIPES

2022

RECIPES TO CLEANSE YOUR BODY AND MIND

MELANIA PILIC

2

Table of Contents

5

10

Artichoke Capers and Artichoke Heart Salad

Ingredients:

1 artichoke, rinsed, patted and shredded

½ cup capers

½ cup artichoke hearts

Dressing

2 tbsp. white wine vinegar

4 tablespoons extra virgin olive oil

Freshly ground black pepper

3/4 cup finely ground almonds

Sea salt

Prep

Combine all of the dressing ingredients in a food processor.

Toss with the rest of the ingredients and combine well.

Mixed Greens Baby Corn and Artichoke Heart Salad

Ingredients:

1 bunch Mesclun, rinsed, patted and shredded

½ cup canned baby corn

½ cup artichoke hearts

Dressing

2 tbsp. white wine vinegar

4 tablespoons extra virgin olive oil

Freshly ground black pepper

3/4 cup finely ground peanuts

Sea salt

Prep

Combine all of the dressing ingredients in a food processor.

Toss with the rest of the ingredients and combine well.

Romaine Lettuce with Tomatillo Dressing

Ingredients:

1 head Romaine lettuce, shredded

4 large tomatoes, seeded and chopped

4 radishes, thinly sliced

Dressing

6 tomatillos, rinsed and halved

1 jalapeno, halved

1 white onion, quartered

2 tablespoons extra virgin olive oil

Kosher salt and freshly ground black pepper

1/2 teaspoon ground cumin

1 cup Dairy free cream cheese

2 tablespoons fresh lemon juice

Prep/Cook

Preheat the oven to 400 degrees F.

For the dressing, place the tomatillos, jalapeno and onion on a cookie sheet.

Drizzle with olive oil and sprinkle with salt and pepper.

Roast in the oven for 25- 30 min. until vegetables begin to brown and slightly darken.

Transfer to a food processor and let it cool then blend.

Add the rest of the ingredients and refrigerate for an hour.

Toss with the rest of the ingredients and combine well.

Greek Romaine Lettuce and Tomato Salad

Ingredients:

1 head romaine lettuce, chopped

4 whole ripe tomatoes, cut into 6 wedges each, then each wedge cut in half

1 whole medium cucumber, peeled, cut into fourths lengthwise, and diced into large chunks

1/2 whole white onion, sliced very thin

30 whole pitted green olives, cut in half lengthwise, plus 6 olives, chopped fine

6 ounces crumbled vegan cheese

Fresh parsley leaves, roughly chopped

Dressing

1/4 cup extra virgin olive oil

2 tablespoons white wine vinegar

1 teaspoon sugar, or more to taste

1 clove garlic, minced

Salt and freshly ground black pepper

Juice of ½ lemon

Sea salt

Prep

Combine all of the dressing ingredients in a food processor and blend.

Season with more salt if necessary.

Toss all of the ingredients together.

Plum Tomato and Cucumber Salad

Ingredients:

5 medium plum tomatoes, halved lengthwise, seeded, and thinly sliced

1/4 white onion, peeled, halved lengthwise, and thinly sliced

1 large cucumber, halved lengthwise and thinly sliced

Dressing

¼ cup extra-virgin olive oil

2 splashes white wine vinegar

Coarse salt and black pepper

Prep

Combine all of the dressing ingredients.

Toss with the rest of the ingredients and combine well.

Enoki Mushroom and Cucumber Salad

Ingredients:

15 Enoki Mushrooms, thinly sliced

1/4 white onion, peeled, halved lengthwise, and thinly sliced

1 large cucumber, halved lengthwise and thinly sliced

Dressing

¼ cup extra-virgin olive oil

2 splashes white wine vinegar

Coarse salt and black pepper

Prep

Combine all of the dressing ingredients.

Toss with the rest of the ingredients and combine well.

Tomato and Zucchini Salad

Ingredients:

5 medium tomatoes, halved lengthwise, seeded, and thinly sliced

1/4 white onion, peeled, halved lengthwise, and thinly sliced

1 large Zucchini halved lengthwise ,thinly sliced & blanched

Dressing

¼ cup extra-virgin olive oil

2 tbsp. apple cider vinegar

Coarse salt and black pepper

Prep

Combine all of the dressing ingredients.

Toss with the rest of the ingredients and combine well.

Tomatillos with Cucumber Salad

Ingredients:

10 Tomatillos, halved lengthwise, seeded, and thinly sliced

1/4 white onion, peeled, halved lengthwise, and thinly sliced

1 large cucumber, halved lengthwise and thinly sliced

Dressing

¼ cup extra-virgin olive oil

2 splashes white wine vinegar

Coarse salt and black pepper

Prep

Combine all of the dressing ingredients.

Toss with the rest of the ingredients and combine well.

Plum Tomato and Onion Salad

Ingredients:

5 medium plum tomatoes, halved lengthwise, seeded, and thinly sliced

1/4 white onion, peeled, halved lengthwise, and thinly sliced

1 large cucumber, halved lengthwise and thinly sliced

Dressing

¼ cup extra-virgin olive oil

2 tbsp. apple cider vinegar

Coarse salt and black pepper

Prep

Combine all of the dressing ingredients.

Toss with the rest of the ingredients and combine well.

Zucchini and tomato Salad

Ingredients:

5 medium tomatoes, halved lengthwise, seeded, and thinly sliced

1/4 white onion, peeled, halved lengthwise, and thinly sliced

1 large Zucchini halved lengthwise ,thinly sliced and blanched

Dressing

¼ cup extra-virgin olive oil

2 splashes white wine vinegar

Coarse salt and black pepper

Prep

Combine all of the dressing ingredients.

Toss with the rest of the ingredients and combine well.

Heirloom Tomato Salad

Ingredients:

3 Heirloom tomatoes, halved lengthwise, seeded, and thinly sliced

1/4 white onion, peeled, halved lengthwise, and thinly sliced

1 large cucumber, halved lengthwise and thinly sliced

Dressing

¼ cup extra-virgin olive oil

2 splashes white wine vinegar

Coarse salt and black pepper

Prep

Combine all of the dressing ingredients.

Toss with the rest of the ingredients and combine well.

Enoki Mushroom Salad

Ingredients:

15 Enoki Mushrooms, thinly sliced

1/4 white onion, peeled, halved lengthwise, and thinly sliced

1 large cucumber, halved lengthwise and thinly sliced

Dressing

¼ cup extra-virgin olive oil

2 tbsp. apple cider vinegar

Coarse salt and black pepper

Prep

Combine all of the dressing ingredients.

Toss with the rest of the ingredients and combine well.

Artichoke Heart and Plum Tomato Salad

Ingredients:

6 Artichoke Hearts (Canned)

5 medium plum tomatoes, halved lengthwise, seeded, and thinly sliced

1/4 white onion, peeled, halved lengthwise, and thinly sliced

1 large cucumber, halved lengthwise and thinly sliced

Dressing

¼ cup extra-virgin olive oil

2 splashes white wine vinegar

Coarse salt and black pepper

Prep

Combine all of the dressing ingredients.

Toss with the rest of the ingredients and combine well.

Baby Corn and Plum Tomato Salad

Ingredients:
½ cup canned baby corn

5 medium plum tomatoes, halved lengthwise, seeded, and thinly sliced

1/4 white onion, peeled, halved lengthwise, and thinly sliced

1 large Zucchini halved lengthwise ,thinly sliced and blanched

Dressing
¼ cup extra-virgin olive oil

2 splashes white wine vinegar

Coarse salt and black pepper

Prep
Combine all of the dressing ingredients.

Toss with the rest of the ingredients and combine well.

Mixed Greens and Tomato Salad

Ingredients:

1 bunch Meslcun, rinsed and drained

5 medium tomatoes, halved lengthwise, seeded, and thinly sliced

1/4 white onion, peeled, halved lengthwise, and thinly sliced

1 large cucumber, halved lengthwise and thinly sliced

Dressing

¼ cup extra-virgin olive oil

2 tbsp. apple cider vinegar

Coarse salt and black pepper

Prep

Combine all of the dressing ingredients.

Toss with the rest of the ingredients and combine well.

Romaine Lettuce and Plum Tomato Salad

Ingredients:

1 bunch Romaine Lettuce, rinsed and drained

5 medium plum tomatoes, halved lengthwise, seeded, and thinly sliced

1/4 white onion, peeled, halved lengthwise, and thinly sliced

1 large cucumber, halved lengthwise and thinly sliced

Dressing

¼ cup extra-virgin olive oil

2 splashes white wine vinegar

Coarse salt and black pepper

Prep

Combine all of the dressing ingredients.

Toss with the rest of the ingredients and combine well.

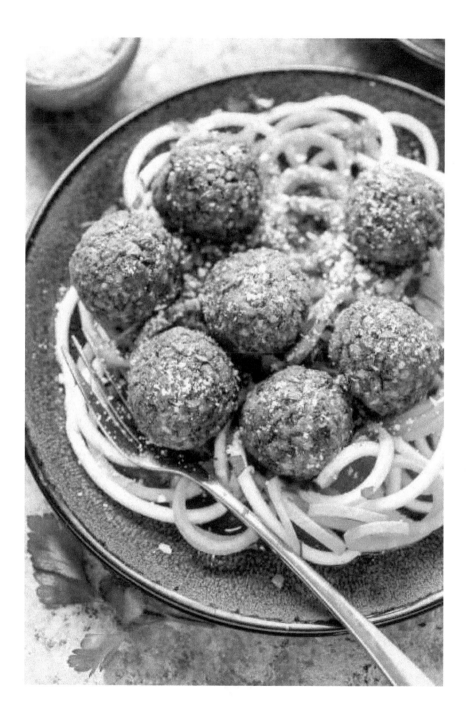

Endive and Enoki Mushroom Salad

Ingredients:

1 bunch Endive, rinsed and drained

15 Enoki Mushrooms, thinly sliced

1/4 white onion, peeled, halved lengthwise, and thinly sliced

1 large cucumber, halved lengthwise and thinly sliced

Dressing

¼ cup extra-virgin olive oil

2 splashes white wine vinegar

Coarse salt and black pepper

Prep

Combine all of the dressing ingredients.

Toss with the rest of the ingredients and combine well.

Artichoke and Tomato Salad

Ingredients:

1 Artichoke, rinsed and drained

5 medium tomatoes, halved lengthwise, seeded, and thinly sliced

1/4 white onion, peeled, halved lengthwise, and thinly sliced

1 large Zucchini halved lengthwise ,thinly sliced and blanched

Dressing

¼ cup extra-virgin olive oil

2 splashes white wine vinegar

Coarse salt and black pepper

Prep

Combine all of the dressing ingredients.

Toss with the rest of the ingredients and combine well.

Kale and Heirloom Tomato Salad

Ingredients:

1 bunch Kale, rinsed and drained

3 Heirloom tomatoes, halved lengthwise, seeded, and thinly sliced

1/4 white onion, peeled, halved lengthwise, and thinly sliced

1 large cucumber, halved lengthwise and thinly sliced

Dressing

¼ cup extra-virgin olive oil

2 tbsp. apple cider vinegar

Coarse salt and black pepper

Prep

Combine all of the dressing ingredients.

Toss with the rest of the ingredients and combine well.

Spinach and Tomatillo Salad

Ingredients:

1 bunch Spinach, rinsed and drained

10 Tomatillos, halved lengthwise, seeded, and thinly sliced

1/4 white onion, peeled, halved lengthwise, and thinly sliced

1 large cucumber, halved lengthwise and thinly sliced

Dressing

¼ cup extra-virgin olive oil

2 splashes white wine vinegar

Coarse salt and black pepper

Prep

Combine all of the dressing ingredients.

Toss with the rest of the ingredients and combine well.

Mesclun and Enoki Mushroom Salad

Ingredients:

1 bunch Meslcun, rinsed and drained

15 Enoki Mushrooms, thinly sliced

1/4 white onion, peeled, halved lengthwise, and thinly sliced

1 large cucumber, halved lengthwise and thinly sliced

Dressing

¼ cup extra-virgin olive oil

2 splashes white wine vinegar

Coarse salt and black pepper

Prep

Combine all of the dressing ingredients.

Toss with the rest of the ingredients and combine well.

Romaine Lettuce and Cucumber Salad

Ingredients:

1 bunch Romaine Lettuce, rinsed and drained

5 medium plum tomatoes, halved lengthwise, seeded, and thinly sliced

1/4 white onion, peeled, halved lengthwise, and thinly sliced

1 large cucumber, halved lengthwise and thinly sliced

Dressing

¼ cup extra-virgin olive oil

2 tbsp. apple cider vinegar

Coarse salt and black pepper

Prep

Combine all of the dressing ingredients.

Toss with the rest of the ingredients and combine well.

Kale Spinach and Zucchini Salad

Ingredients:

1 bunch Kale, rinsed and drained

1 bunch Spinach, rinsed and drained

1/4 white onion, peeled, halved lengthwise, and thinly sliced

1 large Zucchini halved lengthwise ,thinly sliced and blanched

Dressing

¼ cup extra-virgin olive oil

2 splashes white wine vinegar

Coarse salt and black pepper

Prep

Combine all of the dressing ingredients.

Toss with the rest of the ingredients and combine well.

Artichoke Kale and Enoki Mushroom Salad

Ingredients:

1 Artichoke, rinsed and drained

1 bunch Kale, rinsed and drained

15 Enoki Mushrooms, thinly sliced

1/4 white onion, peeled, halved lengthwise, and thinly sliced

1 large cucumber, halved lengthwise and thinly sliced

Dressing

¼ cup extra-virgin olive oil

2 splashes white wine vinegar

Coarse salt and black pepper

Prep

Combine all of the dressing ingredients.

Toss with the rest of the ingredients and combine well.

Endive and Artichoke Salad

Ingredients:

1 bunch Endive, rinsed and drained

1 Artichoke, rinsed and drained

1 large cucumber, halved lengthwise and thinly sliced

Dressing

¼ cup extra-virgin olive oil

2 splashes white wine vinegar

Coarse salt and black pepper

Prep

Combine all of the dressing ingredients.

Toss with the rest of the ingredients and combine well.

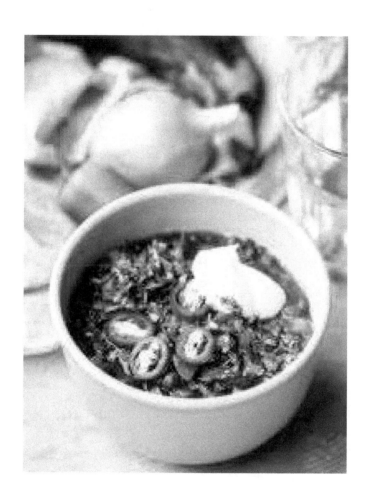

Endive and Zucchini Salad

Ingredients:

1 bunch Romaine Lettuce, rinsed and drained

1 bunch Endive, rinsed and drained

1 large Zucchini halved lengthwise, thinly sliced and blanched

Dressing

¼ cup extra-virgin olive oil

2 splashes white wine vinegar

Coarse salt and black pepper

Prep

Combine all of the dressing ingredients.

Toss with the rest of the ingredients and combine well.

Mesclun and Romaine Lettuce Salad

Ingredients:

1 bunch Meslcun, rinsed and drained

1 bunch Romaine Lettuce, rinsed and drained

1/4 white onion, peeled, halved lengthwise, and thinly sliced

1 large cucumber, halved lengthwise and thinly sliced

Dressing

¼ cup extra-virgin olive oil

2 tbsp. apple cider vinegar

Coarse salt and black pepper

Prep

Combine all of the dressing ingredients.

Toss with the rest of the ingredients and combine well.

Mixed Green and Tomatillo Salad

Ingredients:

1 bunch Meslcun, rinsed and drained

1 bunch Romaine Lettuce, rinsed and drained

10 Tomatillos, halved lengthwise, seeded, and thinly sliced

1/4 white onion, peeled, halved lengthwise, and thinly sliced

1 large Zucchini halved lengthwise ,thinly sliced and blanched

Dressing

¼ cup extra-virgin olive oil

2 splashes white wine vinegar

Coarse salt and black pepper

Prep

Combine all of the dressing ingredients.

Toss with the rest of the ingredients and combine well.

Romaine Lettuce and Endive Salad

Ingredients:

1 bunch Romaine Lettuce, rinsed and drained

1 bunch Endive, rinsed and drained

5 medium plum tomatoes, halved lengthwise, seeded, and thinly sliced

1/4 white onion, peeled, halved lengthwise, and thinly sliced

1 large cucumber, halved lengthwise and thinly sliced

Dressing

¼ cup extra-virgin olive oil

2 splashes white wine vinegar

Coarse salt and black pepper

Prep

Combine all of the dressing ingredients.

Toss with the rest of the ingredients and combine well.

Artichoke and Kale Salad

Ingredients:

1 Artichoke, rinsed and drained

1 bunch Kale, rinsed and drained

3 Heirloom tomatoes, halved lengthwise, seeded, and thinly sliced

1/4 white onion, peeled, halved lengthwise, and thinly sliced

1 large cucumber, halved lengthwise and thinly sliced

Dressing

¼ cup extra-virgin olive oil

2 splashes white wine vinegar

Coarse salt and black pepper

Prep

Combine all of the dressing ingredients.

Toss with the rest of the ingredients and combine well.

Kale and Spinach Salad

Ingredients:

1 bunch Kale, rinsed and drained

1 bunch Spinach, rinsed and drained

15 Enoki Mushrooms, thinly sliced

1/4 white onion, peeled, halved lengthwise, and thinly sliced

1 large cucumber, halved lengthwise and thinly sliced

Dressing

¼ cup extra-virgin olive oil

2 splashes white wine vinegar

Coarse salt and black pepper

Prep

Combine all of the dressing ingredients.

Toss with the rest of the ingredients and combine well.

Carrots and Plum Tomato Salad

Ingredients:

1 cup baby carrots, chopped

5 medium plum tomatoes, halved lengthwise, seeded, and thinly sliced

1/4 white onion, peeled, halved lengthwise, and thinly sliced

1 large cucumber, halved lengthwise and thinly sliced

Dressing

¼ cup extra-virgin olive oil

2 tbsp. apple cider vinegar

Coarse salt and black pepper

Prep

Combine all of the dressing ingredients.

Toss with the rest of the ingredients and combine well.

Corn and Plum Tomato Salad

Ingredients:

1 cup baby corn (canned), drained

5 medium plum tomatoes, halved lengthwise, seeded, and thinly sliced

1/4 white onion, peeled, halved lengthwise, and thinly sliced

1 large Zucchini halved lengthwise ,thinly sliced and blanched

Dressing

¼ cup extra-virgin olive oil

2 splashes white wine vinegar

Coarse salt and black pepper

Prep

Combine all of the dressing ingredients.

Toss with the rest of the ingredients and combine well.

Mixed Green and Baby Carrot Salad

Ingredients:

1 bunch Meslcun, rinsed and drained

1 cup baby carrots, chopped

1 large cucumber, halved lengthwise and thinly sliced

Dressing

¼ cup extra-virgin olive oil

2 splashes white wine vinegar

Coarse salt and black pepper

Prep

Combine all of the dressing ingredients.

Toss with the rest of the ingredients and combine well.

Romaine Lettuce and Baby Corn Salad

Ingredients:

1 bunch Romaine Lettuce, rinsed and drained

1 cup baby corn (canned), drained

1 large cucumber, halved lengthwise and thinly sliced

Dressing

¼ cup extra-virgin olive oil

2 splashes white wine vinegar

Coarse salt and black pepper

Prep

Combine all of the dressing ingredients.

Toss with the rest of the ingredients and combine well.

Baby Corn and Endive Salad

Ingredients:

1 cup baby corn (canned), drained

1 bunch Endive, rinsed and drained

1/4 white onion, peeled, halved lengthwise, and thinly sliced

1 large Zucchini halved lengthwise ,thinly sliced and blanched

Dressing

¼ cup extra-virgin olive oil

2 tbsp. apple cider vinegar

Coarse salt and black pepper

Prep

Combine all of the dressing ingredients.

Toss with the rest of the ingredients and combine well.

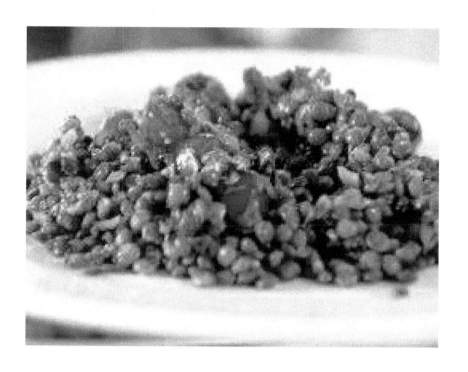

Cauliflower and Tomatillo Salad

Ingredients:

9 cauliflower florets, blanched and drained

10 Tomatillos, halved lengthwise, seeded, and thinly sliced

1/4 white onion, peeled, halved lengthwise, and thinly sliced

1 large cucumber, halved lengthwise and thinly sliced

Dressing

¼ cup extra-virgin olive oil

2 splashes white wine vinegar

Coarse salt and black pepper

Prep

Combine all of the dressing ingredients.

Toss with the rest of the ingredients and combine well.

Broccoli and Tomatillo Salad

Ingredients:

8 broccoli florets, blanched and drained

10 Tomatillos, halved lengthwise, seeded, and thinly sliced

1/4 white onion, peeled, halved lengthwise, and thinly sliced

1 large cucumber, halved lengthwise and thinly sliced

Dressing

¼ cup extra-virgin olive oil

2 splashes white wine vinegar

Coarse salt and black pepper

Prep

Combine all of the dressing ingredients.

Toss with the rest of the ingredients and combine well.

Spinach and Cauliflower Salad

Ingredients:

1 bunch Spinach, rinsed and drained

9 cauliflower florets, blanched and drained

1 large Zucchini halved lengthwise ,thinly sliced and blanched

Dressing

¼ cup extra-virgin olive oil

2 splashes white wine vinegar

Coarse salt and black pepper

Prep

Combine all of the dressing ingredients.

Toss with the rest of the ingredients and combine well.

Kale and Broccoli Salad

Ingredients:

1 bunch Kale, rinsed and drained

8 broccoli florets, blanched and drained

1 large cucumber, halved lengthwise and thinly sliced

Dressing

¼ cup extra-virgin olive oil

2 splashes white wine vinegar

Coarse salt and black pepper

Prep

Combine all of the dressing ingredients.

Toss with the rest of the ingredients and combine well.

Kale Spinach &Broccoli Salad

Ingredients:

1 bunch Kale, rinsed and drained

8 broccoli florets, blanched and drained

1 bunch Spinach, rinsed and drained

Dressing

¼ cup extra-virgin olive oil

2 splashes white wine vinegar

Coarse salt and black pepper

Prep

Combine all of the dressing ingredients.

Toss with the rest of the ingredients and combine well.

Artichoke Kale and Broccoli Salad

Ingredients:

1 Artichoke, rinsed and drained

1 bunch Kale, rinsed and drained

8 broccoli florets, blanched and drained

Dressing

¼ cup extra-virgin olive oil

2 splashes white wine vinegar

Coarse salt and black pepper

Prep

Combine all of the dressing ingredients.

Toss with the rest of the ingredients and combine well.

Baby Corn and Endive Salad

Ingredients:

1 cup baby corn (canned), drained

1 bunch Endive, rinsed and drained

1 Artichoke, rinsed and drained

Dressing

¼ cup extra-virgin olive oil

2 tbsp. apple cider vinegar

Coarse salt and black pepper

Prep

Combine all of the dressing ingredients.

Toss with the rest of the ingredients and combine well.

Mixed Green and Baby Carrot Salad

Ingredients:

1 bunch Meslcun, rinsed and drained

1 cup baby carrots, chopped

1 bunch Romaine Lettuce, rinsed and drained

Dressing

¼ cup extra-virgin olive oil

2 splashes white wine vinegar

Coarse salt and black pepper

Prep

Combine all of the dressing ingredients.

Toss with the rest of the ingredients and combine well.

Tomatillo and Baby Corn Salad

Ingredients:

10 Tomatillos, halved lengthwise, seeded, and thinly sliced

1 cup baby corn (canned), drained

1 bunch Endive, rinsed and drained

1 Artichoke, rinsed and drained

Dressing

¼ cup extra-virgin olive oil

2 splashes white wine vinegar

Coarse salt and black pepper

Prep

Combine all of the dressing ingredients.

Toss with the rest of the ingredients and combine well.

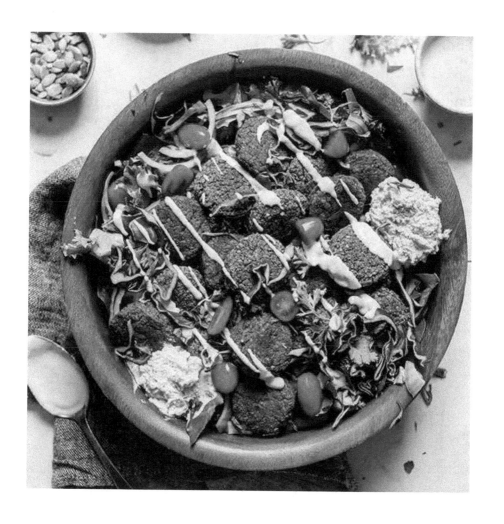

Enoki and Baby Corn Salad

Ingredients:

15 Enoki Mushrooms, thinly sliced

1 cup baby corn (canned), drained

1 bunch Endive, rinsed and drained

1 Artichoke, rinsed and drained

Dressing

¼ cup extra-virgin olive oil

2 tbsp. apple cider vinegar

Coarse salt and black pepper

Prep

Combine all of the dressing ingredients.

Toss with the rest of the ingredients and combine well.

Heirloom Tomato Endive and Artichoke Salad

Ingredients:

3 Heirloom tomatoes, halved lengthwise, seeded, and thinly sliced

1 bunch Endive, rinsed and drained

1 Artichoke, rinsed and drained

1 bunch Kale, rinsed and drained

Dressing

¼ cup extra-virgin olive oil

2 splashes white wine vinegar

Coarse salt and black pepper

Prep

Combine all of the dressing ingredients.

Toss with the rest of the ingredients and combine well.

Kale Plum Tomatoes and Onion Salad

Ingredients:

1 bunch of kale, rinsed and drained

5 medium plum tomatoes, halved lengthwise, seeded, and thinly sliced

1/4 white onion, peeled, halved lengthwise, and thinly sliced

1 large cucumber, halved lengthwise and thinly sliced

Dressing

¼ cup extra-virgin olive oil

2 splashes white wine vinegar

Coarse salt and black pepper

Prep

Combine all of the dressing ingredients.

Toss with the rest of the ingredients and combine well.

Spinach Plum Tomatoes and Onion Salad

Ingredients:

1 bunch of spinach, rinsed and drained

5 medium plum tomatoes, halved lengthwise, seeded, and thinly sliced

1/4 white onion, peeled, halved lengthwise, and thinly sliced

1 large cucumber, halved lengthwise and thinly sliced

Dressing

¼ cup extra-virgin olive oil

2 splashes white wine vinegar

Coarse salt and black pepper

Prep

Combine all of the dressing ingredients.

Toss with the rest of the ingredients and combine well.

Watercress and Zucchini Salad

Ingredients:

1 bunch of watercress, rinsed and drained

5 medium plum tomatoes, halved lengthwise, seeded, and thinly sliced

1/4 white onion, peeled, halved lengthwise, and thinly sliced

1 large Zucchini halved lengthwise ,thinly sliced and blanched

Dressing

¼ cup extra-virgin olive oil

2 tbsp. apple cider vinegar

Coarse salt and black pepper

Prep

Combine all of the dressing ingredients.

Toss with the rest of the ingredients and combine well.

Mangoes tomatoes and Cucumber Salad

Ingredients:

1 cup of cubed mangoes

5 medium plum tomatoes, halved lengthwise, seeded, and thinly sliced

1/4 white onion, peeled, halved lengthwise, and thinly sliced

1 large cucumber, halved lengthwise and thinly sliced

Dressing

¼ cup extra-virgin olive oil

2 splashes white wine vinegar

Coarse salt and black pepper

Prep

Combine all of the dressing ingredients.

Toss with the rest of the ingredients and combine well.

Peaches Tomatoes and Onion Salad

Ingredients:

1 cup of cubed peaches

5 medium tomatoes, halved lengthwise, seeded, and thinly sliced

1/4 white onion, peeled, halved lengthwise, and thinly sliced

1 large cucumber, halved lengthwise and thinly sliced

Dressing

¼ cup extra-virgin olive oil

2 splashes white wine vinegar

Coarse salt and black pepper

Prep

Combine all of the dressing ingredients.

Toss with the rest of the ingredients and combine well.

Black Grapes Tomatillo and White Onion

Ingredients:

12 pcs. black grapes

10 Tomatillos, halved lengthwise, seeded, and thinly sliced

1/4 white onion, peeled, halved lengthwise, and thinly sliced

1 large cucumber, halved lengthwise and thinly sliced

Dressing

¼ cup extra-virgin olive oil

2 splashes white wine vinegar

Coarse salt and black pepper

Prep

Combine all of the dressing ingredients.

Toss with the rest of the ingredients and combine well.

Red Grapes Tomatillo and Zucchini Salad

Ingredients:

10 pcs. red grapes

3 Heirloom tomatoes, halved lengthwise, seeded, and thinly sliced

1/4 white onion, peeled, halved lengthwise, and thinly sliced

1 large Zucchini halved lengthwise ,thinly sliced and blanched

Dressing

¼ cup extra-virgin olive oil

2 splashes white wine vinegar

Coarse salt and black pepper

Prep

Combine all of the dressing ingredients.

Toss with the rest of the ingredients and combine well.

Red Cabbage Plum Tomatoes and Onion Salad

Ingredients:

1/2 medium red cabbage, sliced thinly

5 medium plum tomatoes, halved lengthwise, seeded, and thinly sliced

1/4 white onion, peeled, halved lengthwise, and thinly sliced

1 large cucumber, halved lengthwise and thinly sliced

Dressing

¼ cup extra-virgin olive oil

2 tbsp. apple cider vinegar

Coarse salt and black pepper

Prep

Combine all of the dressing ingredients.

Toss with the rest of the ingredients and combine well.

Napa Cabbage Plum Tomatoes and Cucumber Salad

Ingredients:

1/2 medium Napa cabbage, sliced thinly

5 medium plum tomatoes, halved lengthwise, seeded, and thinly sliced

1/4 white onion, peeled, halved lengthwise, and thinly sliced

1 large cucumber, halved lengthwise and thinly sliced

Dressing

¼ cup extra-virgin olive oil

2 tbsp. apple cider vinegar

Coarse salt and black pepper

Prep

Combine all of the dressing ingredients.

Toss with the rest of the ingredients and combine well.

Red and Napa Cabbage Salad

Ingredients:

1/2 medium red cabbage, sliced thinly

1/2 medium Napa cabbage, sliced thinly

1/4 white onion, peeled, halved lengthwise, and thinly sliced

1 large Zucchini halved lengthwise ,thinly sliced and blanched

Dressing

¼ cup extra-virgin olive oil

2 splashes white wine vinegar

Coarse salt and black pepper

Prep

Combine all of the dressing ingredients.

Toss with the rest of the ingredients and combine well.

Black and Red Grape Salad

Ingredients:

12 pcs. black grapes

10 pcs. red grapes

1/4 white onion, peeled, halved lengthwise, and thinly sliced

1 large cucumber, halved lengthwise and thinly sliced

Dressing

¼ cup extra-virgin olive oil

2 splashes white wine vinegar

Coarse salt and black pepper

Prep

Combine all of the dressing ingredients.

Toss with the rest of the ingredients and combine well.

Mangoes Peaches and Cucumber Salad

Ingredients:

1 cup of cubed mangoes

1 cup of cubed peaches

1/4 white onion, peeled, halved lengthwise, and thinly sliced

1 large cucumber, halved lengthwise and thinly sliced

Dressing

¼ cup extra-virgin olive oil

2 splashes white wine vinegar

Coarse salt and black pepper

Prep

Combine all of the dressing ingredients.

Toss with the rest of the ingredients and combine well.

Watercress Enoki Mushroom and Zucchini Salad

Ingredients:

1 bunch of watercress, rinsed and drained

15 Enoki Mushrooms, thinly sliced

1/4 white onion, peeled, halved lengthwise, and thinly sliced

1 large Zucchini halved lengthwise ,thinly sliced and blanched

Dressing

¼ cup extra-virgin olive oil

2 splashes white wine vinegar

Coarse salt and black pepper

Prep

Combine all of the dressing ingredients.

Toss with the rest of the ingredients and combine well.

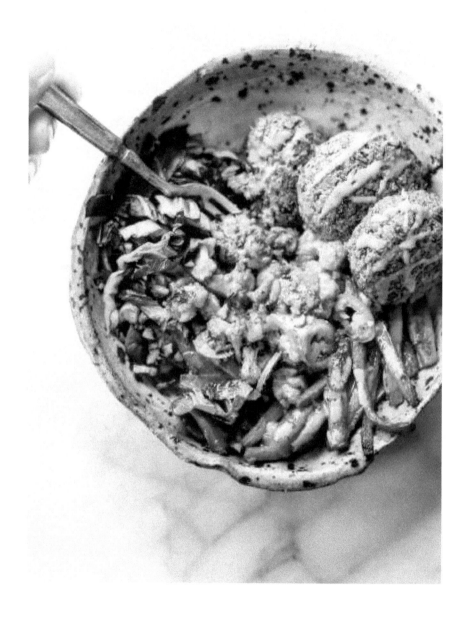

Kale Spinach and Cucumber Salad

Ingredients:

1 bunch of kale, rinsed and drained

1 bunch of spinach, rinsed and drained

1/4 white onion, peeled, halved lengthwise, and thinly sliced

1 large cucumber, halved lengthwise and thinly sliced

Dressing

¼ cup extra-virgin olive oil

2 tbsp. apple cider vinegar

Coarse salt and black pepper

Prep

Combine all of the dressing ingredients.

Toss with the rest of the ingredients and combine well.

Kale Tomato and Zucchini Salad

Ingredients:

1 bunch of kale, rinsed and drained

5 medium plum tomatoes, halved lengthwise, seeded, and thinly sliced

1/4 white onion, peeled, halved lengthwise, and thinly sliced

1 large Zucchini halved lengthwise ,thinly sliced and blanched

Dressing

¼ cup extra-virgin olive oil

2 splashes white wine vinegar

Coarse salt and black pepper

Prep

Combine all of the dressing ingredients.

Toss with the rest of the ingredients and combine well.

Spinach Plum Tomato and Cucumber Salad

Ingredients:

1 bunch of spinach, rinsed and drained

5 medium plum tomatoes, halved lengthwise, seeded, and thinly sliced

1/4 white onion, peeled, halved lengthwise, and thinly sliced

1 large cucumber, halved lengthwise and thinly sliced

Dressing

¼ cup extra-virgin olive oil

2 tbsp. apple cider vinegar

Coarse salt and black pepper

Prep

Combine all of the dressing ingredients.

Toss with the rest of the ingredients and combine well.

Watercress Tomatillo and Cucumber Salad

Ingredients:

1 bunch of watercress, rinsed and drained

10 Tomatillos, halved lengthwise, seeded, and thinly sliced

1/4 white onion, peeled, halved lengthwise, and thinly sliced

1 large cucumber, halved lengthwise and thinly sliced

Dressing

¼ cup extra-virgin olive oil

2 splashes white wine vinegar

Coarse salt and black pepper

Prep

Combine all of the dressing ingredients.

Toss with the rest of the ingredients and combine well.

Mangoes Heirloom Tomatoes and Cucumber Salad

Ingredients:

1 cup of cubed mangoes

3 Heirloom tomatoes, halved lengthwise, seeded, and thinly sliced

1/4 white onion, peeled, halved lengthwise, and thinly sliced

1 large cucumber, halved lengthwise and thinly sliced

Dressing

¼ cup extra-virgin olive oil

2 splashes white wine vinegar

Coarse salt and black pepper

Prep

Combine all of the dressing ingredients.

Toss with the rest of the ingredients and combine well.

Peaches and Tomato Salad

Ingredients:

1 cup of cubed peaches

5 medium tomatoes, halved lengthwise, seeded, and thinly sliced

1/4 white onion, peeled, halved lengthwise, and thinly sliced

1 large cucumber, halved lengthwise and thinly sliced

Dressing

¼ cup extra-virgin olive oil

2 tbsp. apple cider vinegar

Coarse salt and black pepper

Prep

Combine all of the dressing ingredients.

Toss with the rest of the ingredients and combine well.

Black Grapes and Plum Tomato Salad

Ingredients:

12 pcs. black grapes

5 medium plum tomatoes, halved lengthwise, seeded, and thinly sliced

1/4 white onion, peeled, halved lengthwise, and thinly sliced

1 large cucumber, halved lengthwise and thinly sliced

Dressing

¼ cup extra-virgin olive oil

2 splashes white wine vinegar

Coarse salt and black pepper

Prep

Combine all of the dressing ingredients.

Toss with the rest of the ingredients and combine well.

Red Grapes and Zucchini Salad

Ingredients:

10 pcs. red grapes

5 medium plum tomatoes, halved lengthwise, seeded, and thinly sliced

1/4 white onion, peeled, halved lengthwise, and thinly sliced

1 large Zucchini halved lengthwise ,thinly sliced and blanched

Dressing

¼ cup extra-virgin olive oil

2 splashes white wine vinegar

Coarse salt and black pepper

Prep

Combine all of the dressing ingredients.

Toss with the rest of the ingredients and combine well.

Red Cabbage and Tomatillo Salad

Ingredients:

1/2 medium red cabbage, sliced thinly

10 Tomatillos, halved lengthwise, seeded, and thinly sliced

1/4 white onion, peeled, halved lengthwise, and thinly sliced

1 large cucumber, halved lengthwise and thinly sliced

Dressing

¼ cup extra-virgin olive oil

2 splashes white wine vinegar

Coarse salt and black pepper

Prep

Combine all of the dressing ingredients.

Toss with the rest of the ingredients and combine well.

Napa Cabbage Enoki Mushroom and Cucumber Salad

Ingredients:

1/2 medium Napa cabbage, sliced thinly

15 Enoki Mushrooms, thinly sliced

1/4 white onion, peeled, halved lengthwise, and thinly sliced

1 large cucumber, halved lengthwise and thinly sliced

Dressing

¼ cup extra-virgin olive oil

2 tbsp. apple cider vinegar

Coarse salt and black pepper

Prep

Combine all of the dressing ingredients.

Toss with the rest of the ingredients and combine well.

Pineapple Tomato and Cucumber Salad

Ingredients:

1 cup canned pineapple bits

5 medium plum tomatoes, halved lengthwise, seeded, and thinly sliced

1/4 white onion, peeled, halved lengthwise, and thinly sliced

1 large cucumber, halved lengthwise and thinly sliced

Dressing

¼ cup extra-virgin olive oil

2 splashes white wine vinegar

Coarse salt and black pepper

Prep

Combine all of the dressing ingredients.

Toss with the rest of the ingredients and combine well.

Apples Plum Tomatoes and Cucumber Salad

Ingredients:

1 cup Fuji apples cubed

5 medium plum tomatoes, halved lengthwise, seeded, and thinly sliced

1/4 white onion, peeled, halved lengthwise, and thinly sliced

1 large cucumber, halved lengthwise and thinly sliced

Dressing

¼ cup extra-virgin olive oil

2 splashes white wine vinegar

Coarse salt and black pepper

Prep

Combine all of the dressing ingredients.

Toss with the rest of the ingredients and combine well.

Cherries Tomatoes and Onion Salad

Ingredients:

1/4 cup cherries

3 Heirloom tomatoes, halved lengthwise, seeded, and thinly sliced

1/4 white onion, peeled, halved lengthwise, and thinly sliced

1 large Zucchini halved lengthwise ,thinly sliced and blanched

Dressing

¼ cup extra-virgin olive oil

2 splashes white wine vinegar

Coarse salt and black pepper

Prep

Combine all of the dressing ingredients.

Toss with the rest of the ingredients and combine well.

Pickle and Tomato Salad

Ingredients:

1/2 cup pickles

5 medium tomatoes, halved lengthwise, seeded, and thinly sliced

1/4 white onion, peeled, halved lengthwise, and thinly sliced

1 large cucumber, halved lengthwise and thinly sliced

Dressing

¼ cup extra-virgin olive oil

2 splashes white wine vinegar

Coarse salt and black pepper

Prep

Combine all of the dressing ingredients.

Toss with the rest of the ingredients and combine well.

Tomatillo and Corn Salad

Ingredients:

10 Tomatillos, halved lengthwise, seeded, and thinly sliced

1/2 cup canned corn

1 large cucumber, halved lengthwise and thinly sliced

Dressing

¼ cup extra-virgin olive oil

2 tbsp. apple cider vinegar

Coarse salt and black pepper

Prep

Combine all of the dressing ingredients.

Toss with the rest of the ingredients and combine well.

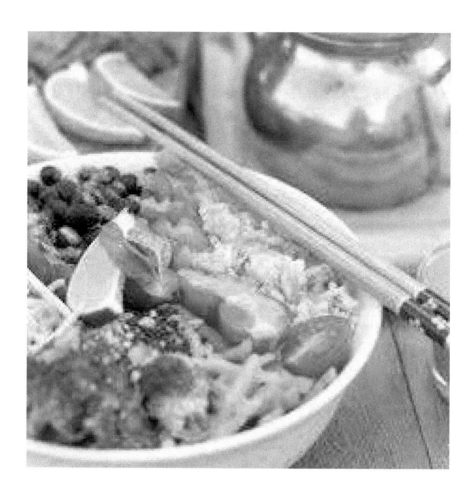

Red Cabbage Artichokes and Cucumber Salad

Ingredients:

1/2 medium red cabbage, sliced thinly

1 cup canned artichokes

1/2 medium Napa cabbage, sliced thinly

1 large cucumber, halved lengthwise and thinly sliced

Dressing

¼ cup extra-virgin olive oil

2 splashes white wine vinegar

Coarse salt and black pepper

Prep

Combine all of the dressing ingredients.

Toss with the rest of the ingredients and combine well.

Corn Red Cabbage and Artichoke Salad

Ingredients:

1/2 cup canned corn

1/2 medium red cabbage, sliced thinly

1 cup canned artichokes

1 large cucumber, halved lengthwise and thinly sliced

Dressing

¼ cup extra-virgin olive oil

2 splashes white wine vinegar

Coarse salt and black pepper

Prep

Combine all of the dressing ingredients.

Toss with the rest of the ingredients and combine well.

Pickles Grapes and Corn Salad

Ingredients:

1/2 cup pickles

10 pcs. red grapes

1/2 cup canned corn

Dressing

¼ cup extra-virgin olive oil

2 splashes white wine vinegar

Coarse salt and black pepper

Prep

Combine all of the dressing ingredients.

Toss with the rest of the ingredients and combine well.

Peaches Cherries and Black Grape Salad

Ingredients:

1 cup of cubed peaches

1/4 cup cherries

12 pcs. black grapes

1/4 white onion, peeled, halved lengthwise, and thinly sliced

1 large cucumber, halved lengthwise and thinly sliced

Dressing

¼ cup extra-virgin olive oil

2 tbsp. apple cider vinegar

Coarse salt and black pepper

Prep

Combine all of the dressing ingredients.

Toss with the rest of the ingredients and combine well.

Pineapple Mangoes and Apple Salad

Ingredients:

1 cup canned pineapple bits

1 cup of cubed mangoes

1 cup Fuji apples cubed

1 large Zucchini halved lengthwise ,thinly sliced and blanched

Dressing

¼ cup extra-virgin olive oil

2 splashes white wine vinegar

Coarse salt and black pepper

Prep

Combine all of the dressing ingredients.

Toss with the rest of the ingredients and combine well.

Kale Spinach and Watercress Salad

Ingredients:

1 bunch of kale, rinsed and drained

1 bunch of spinach, rinsed and drained

1 bunch of watercress, rinsed and drained

Dressing

¼ cup extra-virgin olive oil

2 splashes white wine vinegar

Coarse salt and black pepper

Prep

Combine all of the dressing ingredients.

Toss with the rest of the ingredients and combine well.

Watercress Pineapple and Mangoes Salad

Ingredients:

1 bunch of watercress, rinsed and drained

1 cup canned pineapple bits

1 cup of cubed mangoes

Dressing

¼ cup extra-virgin olive oil

2 tbsp. apple cider vinegar

Coarse salt and black pepper

Prep

Combine all of the dressing ingredients.

Toss with the rest of the ingredients and combine well.

Tomatoes Apples and Peaches Salad

Ingredients:

5 medium tomatoes, halved lengthwise, seeded, and thinly sliced

1 cup Fuji apples cubed

1 cup of cubed peaches

1/4 cup cherries

Dressing

¼ cup extra-virgin olive oil

2 splashes white wine vinegar

Coarse salt and black pepper

Prep

Combine all of the dressing ingredients.

Toss with the rest of the ingredients and combine well.

Enoki Mushroom Corn and Red Cabbage Salad

Ingredients:

15 Enoki Mushrooms, thinly sliced

1/2 cup canned corn

1/2 medium red cabbage, sliced thinly

1 cup canned artichokes

Dressing

¼ cup extra-virgin olive oil

2 splashes white wine vinegar

Coarse salt and black pepper

Prep

Combine all of the dressing ingredients.

Toss with the rest of the ingredients and combine well.

Tomatillos and Apple Salad

Ingredients:

10 Tomatillos, halved lengthwise, seeded, and thinly sliced

1 cup Fuji apples cubed

1 cup of cubed peaches

Dressing

¼ cup extra-virgin olive oil

2 tbsp. apple cider vinegar

Coarse salt and black pepper

Prep

Combine all of the dressing ingredients.

Toss with the rest of the ingredients and combine well.

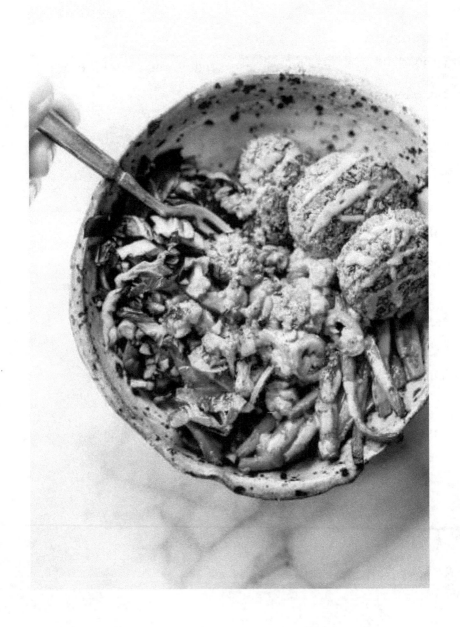

Tomatoes Pickles and Grape Salad

Ingredients:

3 Heirloom tomatoes, halved lengthwise, seeded, and thinly sliced

1/2 cup pickles

10 pcs. red grapes

1/2 cup canned corn

Dressing

¼ cup extra-virgin olive oil

2 splashes white wine vinegar

Coarse salt and black pepper

Prep

Combine all of the dressing ingredients.

Toss with the rest of the ingredients and combine well.

Red Cabbage Artichoke and Cucumber Salad

Ingredients:

1/2 medium red cabbage, sliced thinly

1 cup canned artichokes

1 large cucumber, halved lengthwise and thinly sliced

Dressing

¼ cup extra-virgin olive oil

2 splashes white wine vinegar

Coarse salt and black pepper

Prep

Combine all of the dressing ingredients.

Toss with the rest of the ingredients and combine well.

Pineapple Mango Apple and Cucumber Salad

Ingredients:

1 cup canned pineapple bits

1 cup of cubed mangoes

1 cup Fuji apples cube

1 large cucumber, halved lengthwise and thinly sliced

Dressing

¼ cup extra-virgin olive oil

2 splashes white wine vinegar

Coarse salt and black pepper

Prep

Combine all of the dressing ingredients.

Toss with the rest of the ingredients and combine well.

Artichoke Napa Cabbage and Cucumber Salad

Ingredients:

1 cup canned artichokes

1/2 medium Napa cabbage, sliced thinly

1 large cucumber, halved lengthwise and thinly sliced

Dressing

¼ cup extra-virgin olive oil

2 splashes white wine vinegar

Coarse salt and black pepper

Prep

Combine all of the dressing ingredients.

Toss with the rest of the ingredients and combine well.

Tomatoes Cabbage and Carrot Salad

Ingredients:

3 Heirloom tomatoes, halved lengthwise, seeded, and thinly sliced

1/2 medium Napa cabbage, sliced thinly

5 baby carrots

Dressing

¼ cup extra-virgin olive oil

2 splashes white wine vinegar

Coarse salt and black pepper

Prep

Combine all of the dressing ingredients.

Toss with the rest of the ingredients and combine well.

Napa Cabbage Carrots and Cucumber Salad

Ingredients:

1/2 medium Napa cabbage, sliced thinly

5 baby carrots

1 large cucumber, halved lengthwise and thinly sliced

Dressing

¼ cup extra-virgin olive oil

2 tbsp. apple cider vinegar

Coarse salt and black pepper

Prep

Combine all of the dressing ingredients.

Toss with the rest of the ingredients and combine well.

Roasted Curried Cauliflower

INGREDIENTS

1 head cauliflower , leaves and stems removed and cut into bite-sized florets

1/2 large yellow onion , sliced into thin strips

2 Tbsp extra virgin olive oil

1/2 cup frozen peas

Seasoning ingredients

1/2 Tbsp red curry powder

1/4 tsp crushed red pepper (optional)

Sea salt and pepper to taste

Preheat your oven to 400ºF.

Place the florets in a bowl and rinse under cold water.

Drain the water.

Line a baking pan with foil.

Layer the cauliflower and red onion on the baking sheet.

Pour olive oil and sprinkle the seasoning ingredients.

Combine the ingredients mentioned above thoroughly.

Bake for 45 minutes, stirring once.

Thaw 1/2 cup of peas while the cauliflower is baking.

Remove the cauliflower mixture from the oven after 45 and add the peas.

Toss and coat everything in oil and spices.

Curried Garbanzo Beans

INGREDIENTS

2 Tbsp extra virgin olive oil

1 medium red onion , diced

4 cloves garlic , minced

2 15 oz can garbanzo beans, drained

1 20 oz can tomato sauce

1 cup water

1 Tbsp red curry powder

1/2 bunch fresh cilantro , rinsed and stems removed and coarsely chopped

Stir fry the onion and garlic in a pan with olive oil over medium heat until softened (takes about 4 minutes).

Drain the beans and add to the pan.

Add the tomato sauce, water and curry powder.

Stir everything is well-mixed.

Simmer over medium heat.

Add cilantro to the pot.

Stir and simmer until the sauce has a thick consistency

Brown Lentil Curry

INGREDIENTS

1 Tbsp extra virgin olive oil

3 cloves garlic , minced

1 medium red onion , diced

3 medium carrots (1/2 lb.)

1 cup uncooked brown lentils

2 Tbsp curry powder hot

15 oz can tomato sauce*

Sea salt

1/2 bunch fresh cilantro (optional)

Layer the lentils on a baking pan.

Boil 3 cups of water to a boil in a pot.

Add the lentils.

Boil and turn the heat to low.

Cover and simmer for 20 minutes, or until the lentils become tender.

Drain the lentils.

Stir fry the onion, garlic, and carrots in a pan with olive oil over medium heat until the onions become translucent.

Add curry powder and stir fry for another min.

Add the lentils to the pan, together with the tomato sauce.

Stir and cook through for about 5 minutes.

Season with more salt if necessary.

Garnish with cilantro and serve over rice, naan, pita or crusty bread.

Kale and Tomato Pesto Salad

INGREDIENTS

6 cups kale, finely chopped

15 oz. can white beans, rinsed and drained

1 cup cooked quorn*, chopped

1 cup grape tomatoes, sliced in half

1/2 cup pesto

1 large lemon, cut into wedges

Combine all of the ingredients in a bowl except for the pesto and lemon

Add the pesto and toss until coated.

Garnish with lemon

Slow Cooked Navy Bean Soup

INGREDIENTS

2 Tbsp extra virgin olive oil

6 cloves garlic, minced

1 medium red onion , diced

1/2 lb carrots , sliced thinly into rounds

4 stalks celery (1/2 bunch) ,sliced

1 lb dry navy beans, stones removed, rinsed and drained

1 whole bay leaf

1 tsp dried rosemary

1/2 tsp dried thyme

1/2 tsp Spanish paprika

Freshly cracked pepper (15-20 cranks of a pepper mill)

1 1/2 tsp salt or more to taste

Put the olive oil, garlic, onion, celery, and carrots into slow cooker.

Add the beans ,bay leaf, rosemary, thyme, paprika, and some freshly cracked pepper to the slow cooker.

Add 6 cups of water to the slow cooker and combine the ingredients.

Cover and cook for 8 hours on low or on high for 4 1/2 hours.

Once it's cooked, stir the soup and mash the beans.

Season with more sea salt, if necessary.

Vegan Tofu Wrap

Ingredients

½ red cabbage, shredded

4 heaped tbsp dairy-free yogurt

3 tbsp mint sauce

3 x 200g packs tofu, each cut into 15 cubes

2 tbsp tandoori curry paste

2 tbsp olive oil

2 red onions, sliced

2 large garlic cloves, sliced

8 chapattis

2 limes, cut into quarters

Combine the cabbage, dairy-free yogurt and mint sauce in a bowl.

Season with salt and pepper and set aside.

Combine the tofu ,tandoori paste and 1 tbsp of the oil.

Heat oil on a pan and cook the tofu in batches until golden.

Take the tofu off the pan.

Add the remaining oil, stir fry the onions and garlic, and cook for 9 mins .

Return the tofu to the pan

Add more salt.

To Assemble

Warm the chapattis following package instructions.

Top each one with cabbage, tofu and a squeeze of lime juice.

Vegan Burrito Bowl With Chipotle

Ingredients

125g basmati rice

1 tbsp extra-virgin olive oil

3 garlic cloves, chopped

400g can black beans, drained and rinsed

1 tbsp cider vinegar

1 tsp honey

1 tbsp chipotle paste

100g chopped curly kale

1 avocado halved and sliced

1 medium tomato chopped

1 small yellow onion, chopped

To serve (optional)

chipotle hot sauce

coriander leaves

lime wedges

Cook the rice according to package instructions and keep warm.

In a pan, heat the oil, add the garlic and stir until golden.

Add the beans, vinegar, honey and chipotle.

Season with sea salt

Cook for 2 mins.

Boil the kale for a min. and drain excess moisture.

Divide the rice evenly bet. bowls.

Top with beans, kale, avocado, tomato and onion.

Sprinkle with hot sauce, coriander and lime wedges.

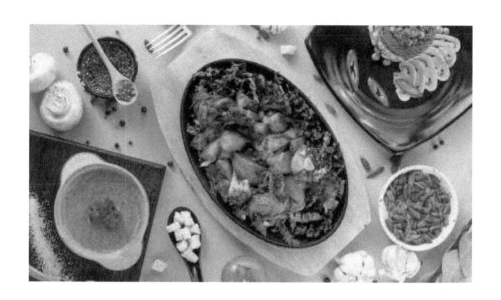

Simplle Vegan Black Bean Chili

Ingredients

2 tbsp extra virgin olive oil

6 garlic cloves, finely chopped

2 large red onions, chopped

3 tbsp sweet pimenton or mild chili powder

3 tbsp ground cumin

Sea salt, to taste

3 tbsp cider vinegar

2 tbsp honey

2 (14 oz.) cans chopped tomatoes

2 (14 oz.) cans black beans, rinsed and drained

For garnishing: crumbled vegan cheese, chopped spring onions, sliced radishes, avocado chunks, soured cream

Heat the olive oil and fry the garlic and onions for until softened.

Stir in the pimenton and cumin, cook for 3 mins,

Add the vinegar, honey, tomatoes and sea salt.

Cook for 10 more mins.

Add the beans and cook for another 10 mins.

Serve with rice and sprinkle with the garnishing ingredients.

Indian Red Lentil and Tomato Stir Fry

Ingredients

200g red lentils, rinsed

2 tbsp olive oil if you're vegan

1 small red onion, finely chopped

4 garlic cloves, finely chopped

Pinch of turmeric

½ tsp garam masala

coriander, to serve

1 small tomato, chopped

Boil the lentils in 1 liter water and a pinch of salt. Bring to a simmer for 25 mins, skimming the bubbles from the top.

Cover and cook for 40 mins, more until thickened.

Heat the oil in a pan over a medium heat.

Stir fry the onion and garlic until the onion softens.

Add the turmeric and garam masala, and cook for another minute.

Place the lentils in a bowl and top with half of the onion mixture.

Garnish with coriander and tomato.

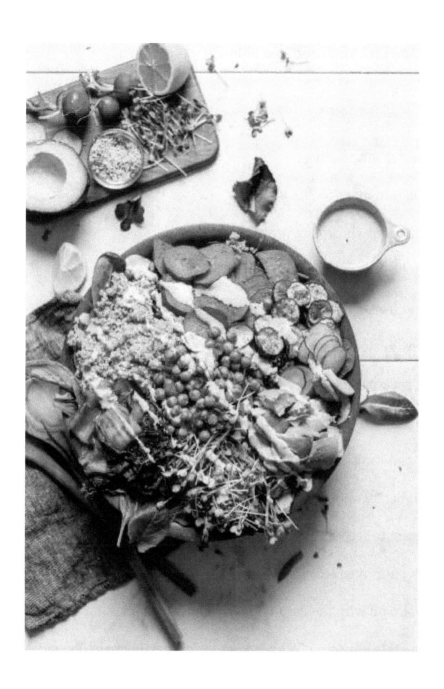

Levantine Chickpea and Pea Salad

Ingredients

½ cup extra virgin olive oil

1 tbsp garam masala

2 (14 oz.) cans chickpeas, drained and rinsed

½ pound ready-to-eat mixed grain pouch

½ pound frozen peas

2 lemons, zested and juiced

1 large pack parsley, leaves roughly chopped

1 large mint leaves, roughly chopped

Half pound radishes, roughly chopped

1 cucumber, chopped

pomegranate seeds, to serve

Preheat your oven to 392 degrees F.

Add ¼ cup oil with the garam masala and add some salt.

Combine this with the chickpeas in a large roasting pan then cook for 15 mins. or until crisp.

Add the mixed grains, peas and lemon zest.

Stir and return to the oven for about 10 mins.

Toss with the herbs, radishes, cucumber, remaining oil and lemon juice.

Season with more salt and garnish with the pomegranate seeds.

Carrot and Cardamom Soup

Ingredients

1 large red onion, finely chopped

4 fat garlic cloves, crushed

1 large carrot, finely chopped

thumb-sized piece of ginger, peeled and finely chopped

2 tbsp olive oil

Pinch of turmeric

Seeds from 10 cardamom pods

1 tsp cumin, seeds or ground

¼ pound red lentils

1 ¾ cup light coconut milk

zest and juice 1 lemon

pinch of chili flakes

handful of parsley, chopped

Heat some oil in a pan and cook the onions, garlic, carrot and ginger until softened.

Add in the turmeric, cardamom and cumin.

Cook for a few mins more, until the spices become aromatic.

Add the lentils, coconut milk, 1 cup of water.

Boil and reduce to a simmer for 15 mins until the lentils become soft.

Process with a hand blender, pulse the soup until it's chunky.

Garnish with lemon zest and juice.

Season with salt, chili and herbs.

Divide among bowls and sprinkle with more lemon zest.

Cauliflower & Basmati Rice Pilaf

Ingredients

1 tbsp olive oil

2 large red onions, sliced

1 tbsp curry paste of your choice

½ pound basmati rice

¾ pound cauliflower florets

1 pound chickpeas, rinsed and drained

2 cups vegetable stock

1/8 cup toasted flaked almonds

handful chopped coriander

Heat the oil in a pan and cook the onions over medium heat for 5 mins until it starts to brown.

Add the curry paste and cook for 1 min.

Add in the rice, cauliflower and chickpeas.

Combine all of this to coat.

Add in the stock and combine thoroughly.

Cover and simmer for 12 ½ mins or until the rice and cauliflower become tender and all the liquid has been reduced.

Add the almonds and coriander.

Vegan Coleslaw Print Recipe

INGREDIENTS

¼ of a large cabbage (375 grams / 13 oz), shredded with a knife or mandolin

1 large carrot, peeled and julienned

½ medium white onion, thinly sliced

Dressing Ingredients

3 tablespoons aquafaba (chickpea cooking liquid)

½ cup canola oil

1 tablespoon apple cider vinegar

2 tablespoons lemon juice

2 tablespoons honey

½ teaspoon sea salt, or more to taste

Combine the vegetables together in a bowl.

In a blender add the aquafaba and slowly drizzle in the oil.

Add the remaining dressing ingredients and blend.

Pour this dressing over the vegetables and toss to combine.

Taste and add salt.

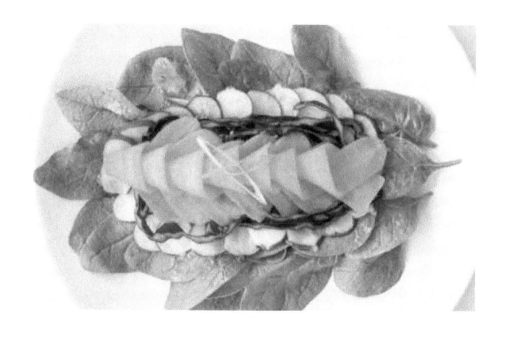

135

Avocado Cream Pasta

Ingredients

2 avocados, pitted and diced

3 cloves garlic, minced

Juice of 1/2 lemon

1/4 cup unsweetened almond milk

1/4 cup water

Sea salt, to taste

Red pepper flakes, to taste

4 halved cherry tomatoes as garnish (optional)

2 cups cooked pasta

Mix the avocados, garlic, and lemon juice in a blender.

Slowly add the almond milk and water to the mixture.

Add sea salt and red pepper flakes.

Toss with your cooked pasta.

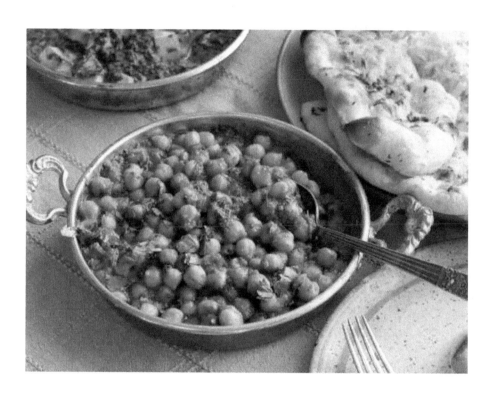

137

Vegan Quorn Salad

16 oz. quorn, cooked

2 tsp. fresh lemon juice

1 stalk celery, diced

1/3 cup minced green onions

1 cup vegan mayonnaise

1 tsp. English mustard

Sea salt and pepper, to taste

Mix the quorn lemon juice, celery, and onions thoroughly.

Add the vegan mayonnaise and the mustard to this mixture.

Season with sea salt and pepper.

Chill and serve.

Vegan Macaroni and Cheese

Ingredients

3 1/2 cups elbow macaroni

1/2 cup vegan margarine

1/2 cup flour

3 1/2 cups boiling water

1-2 tsp. sea salt

2 Tbsp. soy sauce

1 1/2 tsp. garlic powder

Pinch of turmeric

1/4 cup olive oil

1 cup nutritional yeast flakes

Spanish Paprika, to taste

Preheat your oven to 350°F.

Cook the elbow macaroni according to the package instructions.

Drain the noodles.

In a pan, heat the vegan margarine on low until melted.

Add and whisk the flour.

Continue whisking and increase to medium heat until smooth and bubbly.

Add and whisk in the boiling water, salt, soy sauce, garlic powder, and turmeric.

Continue to whisk until dissolved.

Once thick and bubbly, whisk in the oil and the yeast flakes.

Mix 3/4 of the sauce with the noodles and place in a baking dish.

Pour the remaining sauce and season with the paprika.

Bake for 15 minutes.

Broil until crisp for a few min..

Mexican Angel Hair Noodle Soup

5 large tomatoes, cut into large cubes

1 medium red onion, cut into large cubes

3 cloves garlic

2 Tbsp. olive oil

16 oz. angel hair pasta, broken into 1-inch pieces

32 oz. vegetable broth

1/2 tsp. sea salt

1/2 Tbsp. black pepper

2 Tbsp. oregano

2 Tbsp. cumin

Chili flakes, chopped Serrano chilies, or diced jalapeños, to taste (optional)

Cilantro, soy sour cream, and sliced avocado, for garnish (optional)

Puree the tomatoes, red onions, garlic, and oil.

Transfer to a and cook on medium heat.

Add in the noodles, broth, salt, pepper, oregano, and cumin.

Add the chili flakes, Serrano chilies.

Cook for 13 ½ minutes and simmer until the noodles become tender.

Garnish with cilantro, soy sour cream or avocado.

Vegan Pizza

Ingredients

1 piece vegan naan (Indian flatbread)

2 Tbsp. tomato sauce

1/4 cup shredded vegan mozzarella (Daiya brand)

1/4 cup chopped fresh button mushrooms

3 thin tomato slices

2 vegan meatballs Quorn, thawed (if frozen) and cut into small pieces

1 tsp. vegan Parmesan

Pinch of dried basil

Pinch of dried oregano

½ tsp. sea salt

Preheat your oven to 350ºF.

Place the naan on a baking pan.

Layer the sauce evenly over the top and sprinkle with half the vegan mozzarella shreds.

Add in the mushrooms, tomato slices, and vegan meatball pieces.

Layer with the rest of the vegan mozzarella shreds.

Lightly season with the vegan Parmesan, basil, and oregano.

Bake for 25 minutes.

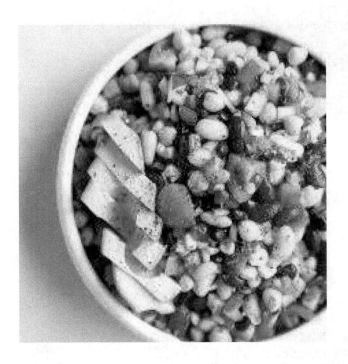

Strawberry and Kale Citrus Salad

Ingredients

1 bunch kale, stemmed and torn to bite sized pieces

1 lb. strawberries, sliced

1/4 cup sliced almonds

Dressing Ingredients

Juice of 1 lemon

3 Tbsp. extra virgin olive oil

1 Tbsp. honey

1/8 tsp. sea salt

1/8 tsp. white pepper

3-4 Tbsp. orange juice

In a bowl combine the kale, strawberries and almonds.

Combine all of the dressing ingredients and pour over the salad.

Makes 3 to 4 servings

Tofu Stir Fry

1 package firm tofu, drained and mashed

Juice of 1/2 lemon

1/2 tsp. salt

1/2 tsp. turmeric

1 Tbsp. extra virgin olive oil

1/4 cup diced green pepper

1/4 cup diced red onion

3 clove garlic, minced

1 Tbsp. chopped flat-leaf parsley

1 Tbsp. vegan bacon bits (optional)

Pepper, to taste (optional)

In a bowl, mix the crumbled tofu, lemon juice, salt, and turmeric thoroughly.

Heat the oil over medium heat and add the pepper, onion, and garlic.

Stir fry for 2 1/2 minutes, or until just softened.

Add the tofu mixture and cook for 15 minutes.

Garnish with the parsley, the soy bacon pieces and pepper.

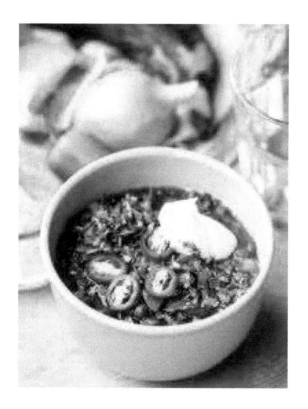

Spinach Stir Fry

1 package firm spinach, rinsed and drained

Juice of 1/2 lemon

1/2 tsp. salt

1/2 tsp. turmeric

1 Tbsp. extra virgin olive oil

1/4 cup diced green pepper

1/4 cup diced red onion

3 clove garlic, minced

1 Tbsp. chopped flat-leaf parsley

1 Tbsp. vegan bacon bits (optional)

Pepper, to taste (optional)

In a bowl, mix the spinach, lemon juice, salt, and turmeric thoroughly.

Heat the oil over medium heat and add the pepper, onion, and garlic.

Stir fry for 2 1/2 minutes, or until just softened.

Add the tofu mixture and cook for 15 minutes.

Garnish with the parsley, the soy bacon pieces and pepper.

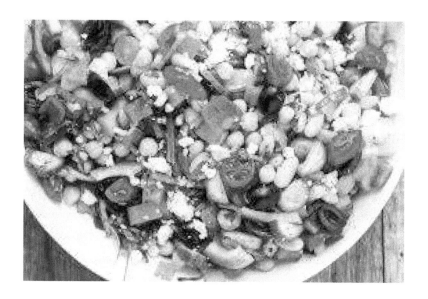

Watercress Stir Fry

1 package firm watercress, rinsed and drained

Juice of 1/2 lemon

1/2 tsp. salt

1/2 tsp. turmeric

1 Tbsp. extra virgin olive oil

1/4 cup diced green pepper

1/4 cup diced red onion

3 clove garlic, minced

1 Tbsp. chopped flat-leaf parsley

1 Tbsp. vegan bacon bits (optional)

Pepper, to taste (optional)

In a bowl, mix the watercress, lemon juice, salt, and turmeric thoroughly.

Heat the oil over medium heat and add the pepper, onion, and garlic.

Stir fry for 2 1/2 minutes, or until just softened.

Add the tofu mixture and cook for 15 minutes.

Garnish with the parsley, the soy bacon pieces and pepper.

Kale Stir Fry

1 package firm kale, rinsed and drained

Juice of 1/2 lemon

1/2 tsp. salt

1/2 tsp. turmeric

1 Tbsp. extra virgin olive oil

1/4 cup diced green pepper

1/4 cup diced red onion

3 clove garlic, minced

1 Tbsp. chopped flat-leaf parsley

1 Tbsp. vegan bacon bits (optional)

Pepper, to taste (optional)

In a bowl, mix the kale, lemon juice, salt, and turmeric thoroughly.

Heat the oil over medium heat and add the pepper, onion, and garlic.

Stir fry for 2 1/2 minutes, or until just softened.

Add the tofu mixture and cook for 15 minutes.

Garnish with the parsley, the soy bacon pieces and pepper.

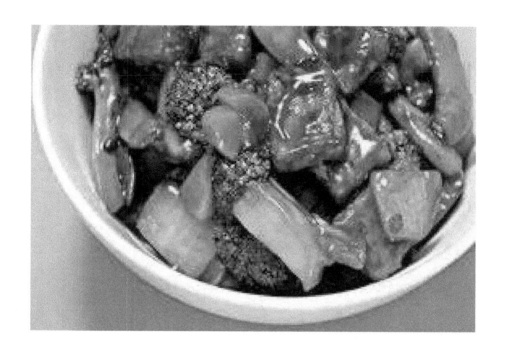

Bok Choy Stir Fry

1 bunch bok choy, rinsed and drained

1/2 tsp. salt

1/2 tsp. turmeric

1 Tbsp. extra virgin olive oil

1/4 cup diced green pepper

1/4 cup diced red onion

3 clove garlic, minced

1 Tbsp. chopped flat-leaf parsley

1 Tbsp. vegan bacon bits (optional)

Pepper, to taste (optional)

In a bowl, mix the bok choy, & salt thoroughly.

Heat the oil over medium heat and add the pepper, onion, and garlic.

Stir fry for 2 1/2 minutes, or until just softened.

Add the tofu mixture and cook for 15 minutes.

Garnish with the parsley , the soy bacon pieces and pepper.

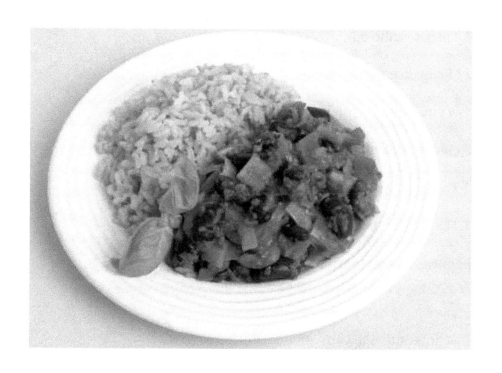

Choy Sum Stir Fry

1 bunch choy sum, rinsed and drained

1/2 tsp.sea salt

1 Tbsp. sesame oil

1/4 cup diced green pepper

1/4 cup diced red onion

3 clove garlic, minced

1 Tbsp. chopped flat-leaf parsley

1 Tbsp. vegan bacon bits (optional)

Pepper, to taste (optional)

In a bowl, mix the choy sum & salt thoroughly.

Heat the oil over medium heat and add the pepper, onion, and garlic.

Stir fry for 2 1/2 minutes, or until just softened.

Add the tofu mixture and cook for 15 minutes.

Garnish with the parsley , the soy bacon pieces and pepper.

Broccoli Stir Fry

20 pcs. broccoli, rinsed, rinsed and drained

Juice of 1/2 lemon

1/2 tsp. salt

1/2 tsp. turmeric

1 Tbsp. extra virgin olive oil

1/4 cup diced green pepper

1/4 cup diced red onion

3 clove garlic, minced

1 Tbsp. chopped flat-leaf parsley

1 Tbsp. vegan bacon bits (optional)

Pepper, to taste (optional)

In a bowl, mix the broccoli, lemon juice, salt, and turmeric thoroughly.

Heat the oil over medium heat and add the pepper, onion, and garlic.

Stir fry for 2 1/2 minutes, or until just softened.

Add the tofu mixture and cook for 15 minutes.

Garnish with the parsley, the soy bacon pieces and pepper.

Vegan Stuffed Crust Pizza

Ingredients

1 box pizza dough (or make your own)

1 block vegan dairy-free mozzarella, cut into strips

1/3 cup vegan pizza sauce

1 medium tomato, thinly sliced

3 fresh basil leaves, coarsely chopped and dipped in olive oil

1 Tbsp. extra virgin olive oil

Preheat your oven to 450°.

Stretch out the pizza dough to your desired thickness and place on a lightly oiled and floured baking sheet.

Place the vegan mozzarella around the edges of the pizza and roll the edges of the dough up over each strip and press down to make a pocket of cheese.

Shred the remaining dairy-free mozzarella.

Spread the pizza sauce over the dough and sprinkle with the shredded vegan cheese.

Garnish with the slices of tomato and basil leaves.

Bake for 20 minutes, or until the crust is nicely browned.

Vegan Alfredo Sauce

1/4 cup vegan margarine

3 cloves garlic, minced

2 cups cooked white beans, rinsed and drained

1 1/2 cups unsweetened almond milk

Sea salt and pepper, to taste

Parsley (optional)

Melt the vegan margarine on low heat.

Add the garlic and cook for 2 ½ minutes.

Transfer to a food processor, add the beans and 1 cup of almond milk.

Blend until smooth.

Pour the sauce to the pan over low heat and season with salt and pepper.

Add the parsley.

Cook until warm.

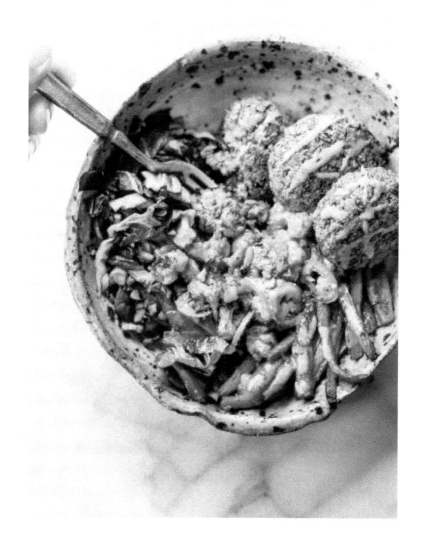

Avocado Salad Sandwich

1 15-oz. can garbanzo beans, rinsed, drained, and skinned

1 large, ripe avocado

1/4 cup chopped fresh cilantro

2 Tbsp. chopped green onions

Juice of 1 lime

Sea salt and pepper, to taste

Bread of your choice

Lettuce

Tomato

Mash the garbanzo beans and avocado with a fork.

Add cilantro , green onions, and lime juice and stir

Season with salt and pepper.

Spread on your favorite bread and garnish with lettuce and tomato

Vegan Fajitas

Ingredients

1 can Refried Beans (15oz)

1 can Pinto Beans (15oz), drained and rinsed

1/4 cup Salsa

1 Red Onion sliced into strips

1 Green Bell Pepper sliced into strips

2 Tbsp Lime Juice

2 tsp Fajita Spice Mix (see below)

Tortillas

Fajita Spice Mix

1 Tbsp. Corn Starch

2 tsp Chili Powder

1 tsp Spanish Paprika

1 tsp honey

1/2 tsp Sea salt

1/2 teaspoon Onion Powder

1/2 teaspoon Garlic Powder

1/2 teaspoon Ground Cumin

1/8 teaspoon Cayenne Pepper

Simmer salsa and refried beans until warm.

Add and mix the fajita spice (leave 2 tsp. behind) mix ingredients in a small bowl.

Sauté the onion, pepper, and 2 tsp of Spice Mix in water and lime juice

Continue until liquid evaporates and vegetables start to brown

Layer the beans in the middle of the tortilla.

Layer with the stir-fried veggies and toppings.

Roll it up and serve.

Butter head Lettuce and Tomato Salad

Ingredients:

8 ounces vegan cheese

6 cups butter head lettuce, 3 bundles, trimmed

1/4 European or seedless cucumber, halved lengthwise, then thinly sliced

3 tablespoons chopped or snipped chives

16 cherry tomatoes

1/2 cup sliced walnuts

1/4 white onion, sliced

2 to 3 tablespoons chopped tarragon leaves

Salt and pepper, to taste

Dressing

1 small shallot, minced

1 tablespoon distilled white vinegar

1/4 lemon, juiced, about 2 teaspoons

1/4 cup extra-virgin olive oil

Prep

Combine all of the dressing ingredients in a food processor.

Toss with the rest of the ingredients and combine well.

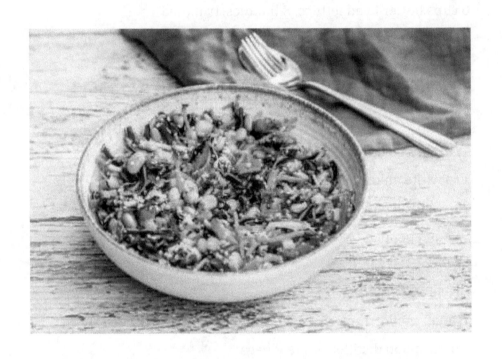

Frisee and Almonds Salad

Ingredients:

8 ounces vegan cheese

6 to 7 cups frisee lettuce, 3 bundles, trimmed

1/4 European or seedless cucumber, halved lengthwise, then thinly sliced

3 tablespoons chopped or snipped chives

16 cherry tomatoes

1/2 cup sliced almonds

1/4 white onion, sliced

2 to 3 tablespoons chopped tarragon leaves

Salt and pepper, to taste

Dressing

1 small shallot, minced

1 tablespoon distilled white vinegar

1/4 lemon, juiced, about 2 teaspoons

1/4 cup extra-virgin olive oil

Prep

Combine all of the dressing ingredients in a food processor.

Toss with the rest of the ingredients and combine well.

Romaine Lettuce and Cashew Salad

Ingredients:

8 ounces vegan cheese

6 to 7 cups romaine lettuce, 3 bundles, trimmed

1/4 European or seedless cucumber, halved lengthwise, then thinly sliced

3 tablespoons chopped or snipped chives

16 cherry tomatoes

1/2 cup sliced cashews

1/4 white onion, sliced

2 to 3 tablespoons chopped rosemary leaves

Salt and pepper, to taste

Dressing

1 small shallot, minced

1 tablespoon distilled white vinegar

1/4 lemon, juiced, about 2 teaspoons

1/4 cup extra-virgin olive oil

Prep

Combine all of the dressing ingredients in a food processor.

Toss with the rest of the ingredients and combine well.

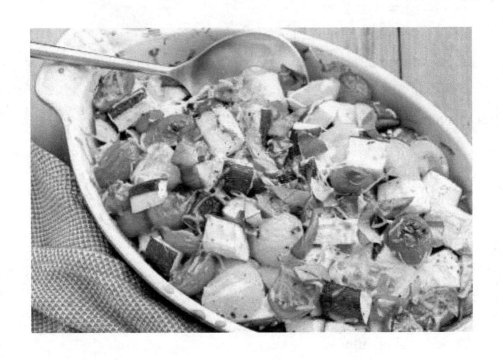

Ice Berg Lettuce and Peanut Salad

Ingredients:

6 to 7 cups iceberg lettuce, 3 bundles, trimmed

1/4 seedless cucumber, halved lengthwise, then thinly sliced

3 tablespoons chopped or snipped chives

16 small tomatoes

1/2 cup peanuts

1/4 vidalla onion, sliced

2 to 3 tablespoons chopped thyme leaves

Salt and pepper, to taste

8 ounces vegan cheese

Dressing

1 small shallot, minced

1 tablespoon distilled white vinegar

1/4 lemon, juiced, about 2 teaspoons

1/4 cup extra-virgin olive oil

½ tsp. English mustard

Prep

Combine all of the dressing ingredients in a food processor.

Toss with the rest of the ingredients and combine well.

Frisee and Walnut Salad

Ingredients:

7 cups frisee lettuce, 3 bundles, trimmed

1/4 cucumber, halved lengthwise, then thinly sliced

3 tablespoons chopped or snipped chives

16 cherry tomatoes

1/2 cup chopped walnuts

1/4 white onion, sliced

2 to 3 tablespoons chopped tarragon leaves

Salt and pepper, to taste

8 ounces vegan cheese

Dressing

1 small green onions , minced

1 tablespoon distilled white vinegar

1/4 lemon, juiced, about 2 teaspoons

1/4 cup extra-virgin olive oil

Prep

Combine all of the dressing ingredients in a food processor.

Toss with the rest of the ingredients and combine well.

Butter head Lettuce and Walnut Salad

Ingredients:

6 to 7 cups butter head lettuce, 3 bundles, trimmed

1/4 European or seedless cucumber, halved lengthwise, then thinly sliced

3 tablespoons chopped or snipped chives

16 cherry tomatoes

1/2 cup sliced walnuts

1/4 red onion, sliced

2 to 3 tablespoons chopped tarragon leaves

Salt and pepper, to taste

8 ounces vegan cheese

Dressing

1 small shallot, minced

1 tablespoon distilled white vinegar

1/4 lemon, juiced, about 2 teaspoons

1/4 cup extra-virgin olive oil

1 tbsp. egg-free mayonnaise

Prep

Combine all of the dressing ingredients in a food processor.

Toss with the rest of the ingredients and combine well.

Romaine Lettuce Cherry Tomatoes and Almond Salad

Ingredients:

6 to 7 cups Romaine lettuce, 3 bundles, trimmed

1/4 European or seedless cucumber, halved lengthwise, then thinly sliced

3 tablespoons chopped or snipped chives

16 cherry tomatoes

1/2 cup sliced almonds

1/4 white onion, sliced

2 tsp. Herbs de Provence

Salt and pepper, to taste

6 ounces vegan cheese

Dressing

1 small shallot, minced

1 tablespoon distilled white vinegar

1/4 lemon, juiced, about 2 teaspoons

1/4 cup extra-virgin olive oil

Prep

Combine all of the dressing ingredients in a food processor.

Toss with the rest of the ingredients and combine well.

Bibb Lettuce Tomatoes and Walnut Salad

Ingredients:

7 cups Bibb lettuce, 3 bundles, trimmed

1/4 European or seedless cucumber, halved lengthwise, then thinly sliced

3 tablespoons chopped or snipped chives

16 cherry tomatoes

1/2 cup sliced walnuts

1/4 white onion, sliced

2 to 3 tablespoons chopped tarragon leaves

Salt and pepper, to taste

8 ounces vegan cheese

Dressing

1 small shallot, minced

1 tablespoon distilled white vinegar

1/4 lemon, juiced, about 2 teaspoons

1/4 cup extra-virgin olive oil

Egg-free mayonnaise

Prep

Combine all of the dressing ingredients in a food processor.

Toss with the rest of the ingredients and combine well.

Boston Lettuce Tomato and Almond Salad

Ingredients:

6 cups Boston lettuce, 3 bundles, trimmed

1/4 European or seedless cucumber, halved lengthwise, then thinly sliced

3 tablespoons chopped or snipped chives

16 cherry tomatoes

1/2 cup sliced almonds

1/4 red onion, sliced

2 to 3 tablespoons chopped tarragon leaves

Salt and pepper, to taste

8 ounces vegan cheese

Dressing

1 small shallot, minced

1 tablespoon distilled white vinegar

1/4 lemon, juiced, about 2 teaspoons

1/4 cup extra-virgin olive oil

1 tsp. Dijon mustard

Prep

Combine all of the dressing ingredients in a food processor.

Toss with the rest of the ingredients and combine well.

Stem Lettuce Cucumber and Almond Salad

Ingredients:

6 to 7 cups stem lettuce, 3 bundles, trimmed

1/4 cucumber, halved lengthwise, then thinly sliced

3 tablespoons chopped or snipped chives

2 mangoes, cubed

1/2 cup sliced almonds

1/4 white onion, sliced

2 to 3 tablespoons chopped tarragon leaves

Salt and pepper, to taste

8 ounces vegan cheese

Dressing

1 small shallot, minced

1 tablespoon distilled white vinegar

1/4 lime, juiced, about 2 teaspoons

1/4 cup extra-virgin olive oil

1 tbsp. honey

1 tsp. English mustard

Prep

Combine all of the dressing ingredients in a food processor.

Toss with the rest of the ingredients and combine well.

Stem Lettuce Cherry Tomatoes and Macadamia Nut Salad

Ingredients:

7 cups stem lettuce, 3 bundles, trimmed

1/4 European or seedless cucumber, halved lengthwise, then thinly sliced

3 tablespoons chopped or snipped chives

16 cherry tomatoes

1/2 cup macadamia nuts

1/4 red onion, sliced

2 to 3 tablespoons fresh thyme

Salt and pepper, to taste

8 ounces vegan cheese

Dressing

1 small shallot, minced

1 tablespoon distilled white vinegar

1/4 lemon, juiced, about 2 teaspoons

1/4 cup extra-virgin olive oil

1 tbsp. honey

1 tsp. Dijon Mustard

Prep

Combine all of the dressing ingredients in a food processor.

Toss with the rest of the ingredients and combine well.

Butter head Lettuce Cherry Tomatoes and Cashew Salad

Ingredients:

7 cups butter head lettuce, 3 bundles, trimmed

1/4 European or seedless cucumber, halved lengthwise, then thinly sliced

3 tablespoons chopped or snipped chives

15 cherry tomatoes

1/2 cup cashews

1/4 white onion, sliced

2 to 3 tablespoons chopped tarragon leaves

Salt and pepper, to taste

8 ounces vegan cheese

Dressing

1 small shallot, minced

1 tablespoon distilled white vinegar

1/4 lemon, juiced, about 2 teaspoons

1/4 cup extra-virgin olive oil

Prep

Combine all of the dressing ingredients in a food processor.

Toss with the rest of the ingredients and combine well.

Romaine Lettuce Cherry Tomatoes and Macadamia Nut Salad

Ingredients:

6 ½ cups romaine lettuce, 3 bundles, trimmed

1/4 European or seedless cucumber, halved lengthwise, then thinly sliced

3 tablespoons chopped or snipped chives

16 cherry tomatoes

1/2 cup macadamia nuts

1/4 white onion, sliced

2 to 3 tablespoons chopped tarragon leaves

Salt and pepper, to taste

8 ounces vegan cheese

Dressing

1 small shallot, minced

1 tablespoon distilled white vinegar

1/4 lemon, juiced, about 2 teaspoons

1/4 cup extra-virgin olive oil

Prep

Combine all of the dressing ingredients in a food processor.

Toss with the rest of the ingredients and combine well.

Iceberg Lettuce Apples and Walnut Salad

Ingredients:

8 ounces vegan cheese

6 to 7 cups iceberg lettuce, 3 bundles, trimmed

1/4 European or seedless cucumber, halved lengthwise, then thinly sliced

3 tablespoons chopped or snipped chives

2 apples, cored and cubed into 2 inch cubes

1/2 cup sliced walnuts

1/4 white onion, sliced

2 to 3 tablespoons chopped tarragon leaves

Salt and pepper, to taste

Dressing

1 small shallot, minced

2 tablespoons distilled white vinegar

1/4 cup sesame oil

1 teaspoon honey

½ tsp. egg-free mayonnaise

Prep

Combine all of the dressing ingredients in a food processor.

Toss with the rest of the ingredients and combine well.

Lettuce Tomatoes and Almond Salad

Ingredients:

8 ounces vegan cheese

7 cups loose leaf lettuce, 3 bundles, trimmed

1/4 European or seedless cucumber, halved lengthwise, then thinly sliced

3 tablespoons chopped or snipped chives

16 cherry tomatoes

1/2 cup sliced almonds

1/4 red onion, sliced

2 to 3 tablespoons chopped thyme

Salt and pepper, to taste

Dressing

1 small shallot, minced

1 tablespoon distilled white vinegar

1/4 lemon, juiced, about 2 teaspoons

1/4 cup extra-virgin olive oil

1 tbsp. egg free mayonnaise

Prep

Combine all of the dressing ingredients in a food processor.

Toss with the rest of the ingredients and combine well.

Frisee Cherries and Macadamia Nut Salad

Ingredients:

6 to 7 cups frisee lettuce, 3 bundles, trimmed

1/4 European or seedless cucumber, halved lengthwise, then thinly sliced

3 tablespoons chopped or snipped chives

16 cherries, pitted

1/2 cup macadamia nuts

1/4 red onion, sliced

2 to 3 tablespoons chopped tarragon leaves

Sea salt and pepper, to taste

8 ounces vegan cheese

Dressing

1 tbsp. chives, snipped

1 tablespoon distilled white vinegar

1/4 lemon, juiced, about 2 teaspoons

1/4 cup extra-virgin olive oil

1 tbsp. honey

Prep

Combine all of the dressing ingredients in a food processor.

Toss with the rest of the ingredients and combine well.

Romaine Lettuce Grapes and Walnut Salad

Ingredients:

7 loose romaine lettuce, 3 bundles, trimmed

1/4 cucumber, halved lengthwise, then thinly sliced

4 tablespoons chopped or snipped chives

16 grapes

1/2 cup sliced walnuts

1/4 white onion, sliced

Salt and pepper, to taste

Dressing

2 tablespoons distilled white vinegar

1/4 cup sesame oil

1 tsp. hoi sin sauce

Prep

Combine all of the dressing ingredients in a food processor.

Toss with the rest of the ingredients and combine well.

Butter Lettuce Cherry Tomatoes and Thai Basil Salad

Ingredients:

6 to 7 cups butter lettuce, 3 bundles, trimmed

1/4 European or seedless cucumber, halved lengthwise, then thinly sliced

3 tablespoons chopped or snipped chives

16 cherry tomatoes

1/2 cup walnuts

1/4 white onion, sliced

2 to 3 tablespoons chopped Thai basil

Salt and pepper, to taste

Dressing

1 small scallions, minced

1 tablespoon distilled white vinegar

1/4 cup sesame oil

1 tbsp. sambal oelek

Prep

Combine all of the dressing ingredients in a food processor.

Toss with the rest of the ingredients and combine well.

Smoky Lettuce and Tarragon Salad

Ingredients:

8 ounces vegan cheese

6 to 7 cups loose leaf lettuce, 3 bundles, trimmed

1/4 European or seedless cucumber, halved lengthwise, then thinly sliced

3 tablespoons chopped or snipped chives

16 cherry tomatoes

1/2 cup sliced almonds

1/4 white onion, sliced

2 to 3 tablespoons chopped tarragon leaves

Salt and pepper, to taste

Dressing

1 tsp. cumin

1 tsp. annatto seeds

1 /2 tsp. cayenne pepper

1 tablespoon distilled white vinegar

1/4 lime, juiced, about 2 teaspoons

1/4 cup extra-virgin olive oil

Prep

Combine all of the dressing ingredients in a food processor.

Toss with the rest of the ingredients and combine well.

Lettuce Mint Leaves and Cashew Salad

Ingredients:

6 to 7 cups loose leaf lettuce, 3 bundles, trimmed

1/4 European or seedless cucumber, halved lengthwise, then thinly sliced

3 tablespoons chopped or snipped chives

16 grapes

1/2 cup cashews

1/4 red onion, sliced

2 to 3 tablespoons chopped mint leaves

Salt and pepper, to taste

8 ounces vegan cheese

Dressing

1 small shallot, minced

1 tablespoon distilled white vinegar

1/4 lime, juiced, about 2 teaspoons

1/4 cup extra-virgin olive oil

1 tsp. honey

 Prep

Combine all of the dressing ingredients in a food processor.

 Toss with the rest of the ingredients and combine well.

Lettuce Tomatoes and Peanut Salad

Ingredients:

6 to 7 cups romaine lettuce, 3 bundles, trimmed

1/4 European or seedless cucumber, halved lengthwise, then thinly sliced

3 tablespoons chopped or snipped chives

16 cherry tomatoes

1/2 cup sliced peanuts

1/4 yellow onion, sliced

Salt and pepper, to taste

8 ounces vegan cheese

Dressing

1 small shallot, minced

1 tablespoon distilled white vinegar

1/4 lemon, juiced, about 2 teaspoons

1/4 cup extra-virgin olive oil

Prep

Combine all of the dressing ingredients in a food processor.

Toss with the rest of the ingredients and combine well.

Butter head Lettuce Orange and Almond Salad

Ingredients:

6 to 7 cups Butter head lettuce, 3 bundles, trimmed

1/4 cucumber, halved lengthwise, then thinly sliced

3 tablespoons chopped or snipped mint leaves

8 slices of mandarin oranges, skins removed and sliced in half

1/2 cup sliced almonds

1/4 white onion, sliced

Salt and pepper, to taste

8 ounces vegan cheese

Dressing

1 small shallot, minced

1 tablespoon distilled white vinegar

1/4 lime, juiced, about 2 teaspoons

1/4 cup sesame oil

1 tbsp. honey

Prep

Combine all of the dressing ingredients in a food processor.

Toss with the rest of the ingredients and combine well.

Simple Lettuce Tomatoes and Almond Salad

Ingredients:

6 to 7 cups Iceberg lettuce, 3 bundles, trimmed

1/4 European or seedless cucumber, halved lengthwise, then thinly sliced

3 tablespoons chopped or snipped chives

16 cherry tomatoes

1/2 cup sliced almonds

1/4 red onion, sliced

2 sprigs of fresh rosemary

Salt and pepper, to taste

8 ounces vegan cheese

Dressing

1 small scallions, minced

1 tablespoon distilled white vinegar

1/4 lemon, juiced, about 2 teaspoons

1/4 cup extra-virgin olive oil

1 egg-free mayonnaise

Prep

Combine all of the dressing ingredients in a food processor.

Toss with the rest of the ingredients and combine well.

Romaine Lettuce Tomatoes & Hazelnut Salad

Ingredients:

6 to 7 cups Romaine lettuce, 3 bundles, trimmed

1/4 European or seedless cucumber, halved lengthwise, then thinly sliced

3 tablespoons chopped or snipped chives

16 cherry tomatoes

1/2 cup hazelnuts

10 black grapes, seedless

2 to 3 tablespoons chopped tarragon leaves

Salt and pepper, to taste

8 ounces vegan cheese

Dressing

1 small shallot, minced

1 tablespoon distilled white vinegar

1/4 lemon, juiced, about 2 teaspoons

1/4 cup extra-virgin olive oil

1 tbsp. honey

Prep

Combine all of the dressing ingredients in a food processor.

Toss with the rest of the ingredients and combine well.

Frisee Lettuce Onion and Tarragon Salad

Ingredients:

8 ounces vegan cheese

6 to 7 cups frisee lettuce, 3 bundles, trimmed

1/4 European or seedless cucumber, halved lengthwise, then thinly sliced

3 tablespoons chopped or snipped chives

16 cherry tomatoes

1/2 cup sliced almonds

1/4 white onion, sliced

2 to 3 tablespoons chopped tarragon leaves

Salt and pepper, to taste

Dressing

1 small shallot, minced

1 tablespoon distilled white vinegar

1/4 lemon, juiced, about 2 teaspoons

1/4 cup extra-virgin olive oil

Prep

Combine all of the dressing ingredients in a food processor.

Toss with the rest of the ingredients and combine well.

Frisee Tomatoes Almond and Tarragon Salad

Ingredients:

8 ounces vegan cheese

6 to 7 cups frisee lettuce, 3 bundles, trimmed

1/4 European or seedless cucumber, halved lengthwise, then thinly sliced

3 tablespoons chopped or snipped chives

16 cherry tomatoes

1/2 cup sliced almonds

1/4 white onion, sliced

2 to 3 tablespoons chopped tarragon leaves

Salt and pepper, to taste

Dressing

1 small shallot, minced

1 tablespoon distilled white vinegar

1/4 lemon, juiced, about 2 teaspoons

1/4 cup extra-virgin olive oil

Prep

Combine all of the dressing ingredients in a food processor.

Toss with the rest of the ingredients and combine well.

Frisee Tomatoes and Hazelnut Salad

Ingredients:

8 ounces vegan cheese

6 to 7 cups frisee lettuce, 3 bundles, trimmed

1/4 European or seedless cucumber, halved lengthwise, then thinly sliced

3 tablespoons chopped or snipped chives

16 cherry tomatoes

1/2 cup sliced hazelnuts

1/4 white onion, sliced

2 to 3 tablespoons chopped tarragon leaves

Salt and pepper, to taste

Dressing

1 small shallot, minced

1 tablespoon distilled white vinegar

1/4 lemon, juiced, about 2 teaspoons

1/4 cup extra-virgin olive oil

Prep

Combine all of the dressing ingredients in a food processor.

Toss with the rest of the ingredients and combine well.

Frisee and Zucchini Salad

Ingredients:

8 ounces vegan cheese

6 to 7 cups frisee lettuce, 3 bundles, trimmed

1/4 Zucchini, halved lengthwise, then thinly sliced

16 cherry tomatoes

1/2 cup sliced almonds

1/4 white onion, sliced

2 to 3 tablespoons chopped tarragon leaves

Salt and pepper, to taste

Dressing

1 small shallot, minced

1 tablespoon distilled white vinegar

1/4 lemon, juiced, about 2 teaspoons

1/4 cup extra-virgin olive oil

Prep

Combine all of the dressing ingredients in a food processor.

Toss with the rest of the ingredients and combine well.

Romaine Lettuce and Hazelnut Salad

Ingredients:

8 ounces vegan cheese

6 to 7 cups Romaine lettuce, 3 bundles, trimmed

1/4 European or seedless cucumber, halved lengthwise, then thinly sliced

3 tablespoons chopped or snipped chives

16 cherry tomatoes

1/2 cup sliced hazelnuts

1/4 white onion, sliced

2 to 3 tablespoons chopped tarragon leaves

Salt and pepper, to taste

Dressing

1 small shallot, minced

1 tablespoon distilled white vinegar

1/4 lemon, juiced, about 2 teaspoons

1/4 cup extra-virgin olive oil

Prep

Combine all of the dressing ingredients in a food processor.

Toss with the rest of the ingredients and combine well.

Iceberg Lettuce Tomatoes and Almond Salad

Ingredients:

8 ounces vegan cheese

6 to 7 cups Iceberg lettuce, 3 bundles, trimmed

1/4 European or seedless cucumber, halved lengthwise, then thinly sliced

3 tablespoons chopped or snipped chives

16 cherry tomatoes

1/2 cup sliced almonds

1/4 white onion, sliced

2 to 3 tablespoons chopped tarragon leaves

Salt and pepper, to taste

Dressing

1 small shallot, minced

1 tablespoon distilled white vinegar

1/4 lemon, juiced, about 2 teaspoons

1/4 cup extra-virgin olive oil

Prep

Combine all of the dressing ingredients in a food processor.

Toss with the rest of the ingredients and combine well.

Frisee and Feta Salad

Ingredients:

6 to 7 cups butter head lettuce, 3 bundles, trimmed

1/4 seedless cucumber, halved lengthwise, then thinly sliced

3 tablespoons chopped or snipped chives

16 cherry tomatoes

1/2 cup pistachios

1/4 white onion, sliced

2 to 3 tablespoons chopped tarragon leaves

Salt and pepper, to taste

8 ounces vegan cheese

Dressing

1 small shallot, minced

1 tablespoon distilled white vinegar

1/4 lemon, juiced, about 2 teaspoons

1/4 cup extra-virgin olive oil

1 tbsp. pesto sauce

Prep

Combine all of the dressing ingredients in a food processor.

Toss with the rest of the ingredients and combine well.

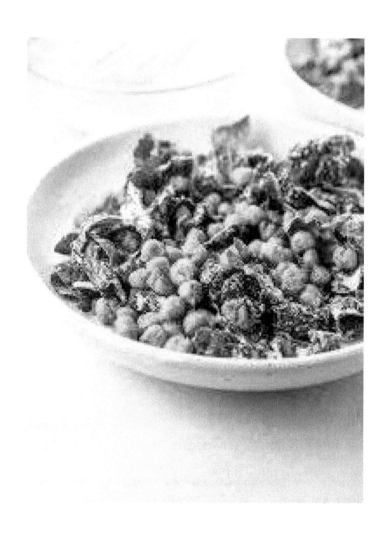

Frisee and Feta Salad

Ingredients:

6 to 7 cups romaine lettuce, 3 bundles, trimmed

1/4 European or seedless cucumber, halved lengthwise, then thinly sliced

3 tablespoons chopped or snipped chives

16 cherry tomatoes

1/2 cup macadamia nuts

1/4 red onion, sliced

Salt and pepper, to taste

5 ounces vegan cheese

Dressing

1 small shallot, minced

1 tablespoon distilled white vinegar

1/4 lemon, juiced, about 2 teaspoons

1/4 cup extra-virgin olive oil

1 tbsp. pesto sauce

Prep

Combine all of the dressing ingredients in a food processor.

Toss with the rest of the ingredients and combine well.

Lettuce Basil and Vegan Cheese

Ingredients:

6 to 7 cups loose leaf lettuce, 3 bundles, trimmed

1/4 cucumber, halved lengthwise, then thinly sliced

16 cherry tomatoes

1/4 red onion, sliced

2 to 3 tablespoons chopped fresh basil

Salt and pepper, to taste

8 ounces vegan cheese

Dressing

1 small shallot, minced

1 tablespoon distilled white vinegar

1/4 lemon, juiced, about 2 teaspoons

1/4 cup extra-virgin olive oil

Prep

Combine all of the dressing ingredients in a food processor.

Toss with the rest of the ingredients and combine well.

Romaine Lettuce and Pistachio Salad

Ingredients:

8 ounces vegan cheese

6 to 7 cups Romaine lettuce, 3 bundles, trimmed

1/4 European or seedless cucumber, halved lengthwise, then thinly sliced

3 tablespoons chopped or snipped chives

16 cherry tomatoes

1/2 cup sliced pistachios

1/4 Vidalla onion, sliced

2 to 3 tablespoons chopped tarragon leaves

Salt and pepper, to taste

Dressing

1 small shallot, minced

1 tablespoon distilled white vinegar

1/4 lemon, juiced, about 2 teaspoons

1/4 cup extra-virgin olive oil

Prep

Combine all of the dressing ingredients in a food processor.

Toss with the rest of the ingredients and combine well.

Frisee Lettuce Tomatoes and Onion in Macadamia Nut Oil Vinaigrette

Ingredients:

6 to 7 cups frisee lettuce, 3 bundles, trimmed

1/4 cucumber, halved lengthwise, then thinly sliced

3 tablespoons chopped or snipped chives

16 cherry tomatoes

1/2 cup sliced almonds

1/4 red onion, sliced

2 to 3 tablespoons chopped parsley

Salt and pepper, to taste

8 ounces vegan cheese

Dressing

1 small scallions, minced

1 tablespoon distilled white vinegar

1/4 lemon, juiced, about 2 teaspoons

1/4 cup macadamia nut oil

Prep

Combine all of the dressing ingredients in a food processor.

Toss with the rest of the ingredients and combine well.

Romaine Lettuce Tomatoes and Pistachios

Ingredients:

8 ounces vegan cheese

6 to 7 cups romaine lettuce, 3 bundles, trimmed

1/4 European or seedless cucumber, halved lengthwise, then thinly sliced

3 tablespoons chopped or snipped chives

16 cherry tomatoes

1/2 cup pistachios

1/4 red onion, sliced

Salt and pepper, to taste

Dressing

1 small shallot, minced

1 tablespoon distilled white vinegar

1/4 lemon, juiced, about 2 teaspoons

1/4 cup extra-virgin olive oil

Prep

Combine all of the dressing ingredients in a food processor.

Toss with the rest of the ingredients and combine well.

Grilled Kale and Green Bean Salad

Ingredients:

8 pcs. Green Beans

1 bunch of kale, rinsed and drained

¼ cup extra virgin olive oil

Dressing

2 tbsp. macadamia nut oil

Steak seasoning, McCormick

3 tbsp. dry sherry

1 tbsp. dried thyme

Prep

Preheat the grill to medium high.

Brush the vegetable with ¼ cup oil.

Cook

Sprinkle with salt and pepper and grill for 4 min. per side.

Flip once only so you can get the grill marks on the vegetable.

Combine all of the dressing ingredients.

Drizzle over the vegetable.

Grilled Green Bean and Cauliflower Salad

Ingredients:

8 pcs. Green Beans

7 Broccoli florets

12 ounces eggplant (about 12 ounces total), sliced lengthwise into 1/2-inch-thick rectangles

4 large Tomatoes, sliced thick

5 Cauliflower florets

¼ cup macadamia nut oil

Dressing Ingredients

6 tbsp. extra virgin olive oil

Sea salt, to taste

3 tbsp. apple cider vinegar

1 tbsp. honey

1 tsp. Egg-free mayonnaise

Prep

Preheat the grill to medium high.

Brush the vegetable with ¼ cup oil.

Cook

Sprinkle with salt and pepper and grill for 4 min. per side.

Flip once only so you can get the grill marks on the vegetable.

Combine all of the dressing ingredients.

Drizzle over the vegetable.

Grilled Eggplant Carrots and Watercress Salad

Ingredients:

12 ounces eggplant (about 12 ounces total), sliced lengthwise into 1/2-inch-thick rectangles

5 baby carrots

1 bunch of watercress, rinsed and drained1 bunch endives

1/4 cup extra virgin olive oil

Dressing Ingredients

6 tbsp. olive oil

3 dashes of Tabasco hot sauce

Sea salt, to taste

3 tbsp. white wine vinegar

1 tsp. Egg-free mayonnaise

Prep

Preheat the grill to medium high.

Brush the vegetable with ¼ cup oil.

Cook

Sprinkle with salt and pepper and grill for 4 min. per side.

Flip once only so you can get the grill marks on the vegetable.

Combine all of the dressing ingredients.

Drizzle over the vegetable.

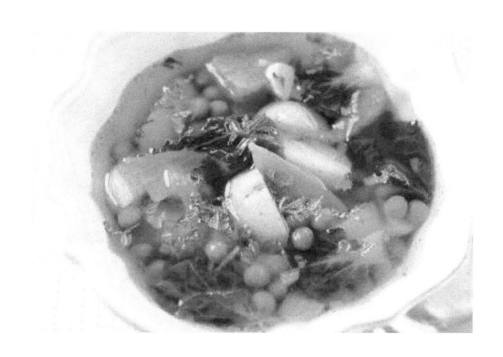

Grilled Carrots Endives and Watercress Salad

Ingredients:

5 baby carrots

1 bunch of watercress, rinsed and drained

1 bunch endives

1/4 cup extra virgin olive oil

Dressing Ingredients

6 tbsp. extra virgin olive oil

Sea salt, to taste

3 tbsp. apple cider vinegar

1 tbsp. honey

1 tsp. Egg-free mayonnaise

Prep

Preheat the grill to medium high.

Brush the vegetable with ¼ cup oil.

Cook

Sprinkle with salt and pepper and grill for 4 min. per side.

Flip once only so you can get the grill marks on the vegetable.

Combine all of the dressing ingredients.

Drizzle over the vegetable.

Grilled Eggplant and Baby Carrot Salad

Ingredients:

12 ounces eggplant (about 12 ounces total), sliced lengthwise into 1/2-inch-thick rectangles

5 baby carrots

1 bunch of watercress, rinsed and drained

1/4 cup extra virgin olive oil

Dressing Ingredients

4 tbsp. olive oil

Steak seasoning, McCormick

2 tbsp. white vinegar

1 tbsp. dried thyme

1/2 tsp. sea salt

Prep

Preheat the grill to medium high.

Brush the vegetable with ¼ cup oil.

Cook

Sprinkle with salt and pepper and grill for 4 min. per side.

Flip once only so you can get the grill marks on the vegetable.

Combine all of the dressing ingredients.

Drizzle over the vegetable.

CPSIA information can be obtained
at www.ICGtesting.com
Printed in the USA
LVHW051057080622
720760LV00012B/1040

9 781804 506899